Daniel José Olazabal Guerra

Informational competencies in health technology students

Daniel José Olazabal Guerra

Informational competencies in health technology students

Towards a proposed methodological strategy

ScienciaScripts

Imprint

Any brand names and product names mentioned in this book are subject to trademark, brand or patent protection and are trademarks or registered trademarks of their respective holders. The use of brand names, product names, common names, trade names, product descriptions etc. even without a particular marking in this work is in no way to be construed to mean that such names may be regarded as unrestricted in respect of trademark and brand protection legislation and could thus be used by anyone.

Cover image: www.ingimage.com

This book is a translation from the original published under ISBN 978-613-9-41225-9.

Publisher:
Sciencia Scripts
is a trademark of
Dodo Books Indian Ocean Ltd. and OmniScriptum S.R.L publishing group

120 High Road, East Finchley, London, N2 9ED, United Kingdom
Str. Armeneasca 28/1, office 1, Chisinau MD-2012, Republic of Moldova, Europe
Printed at: see last page
ISBN: 978-620-7-94841-3

INFORMATIONAL COMPETENCIES IN HEALTH TECHNOLOGY STUDENTS.

Towards a Methodological Strategy proposal.

Daniel José Olazabal Guerra

2024

THINKING

"In times of change, those who are open to learning will own the future, while those who think they know it all will be well equipped for a world that no longer exists."

Eric Hoffner.

SUMMARY

Information and Communication Technologies are nowadays an important working tool to dynamize the process of scientific research at all levels. Currently, digital competencies promote knowledge societies, students and teachers should understand their presence in the various virtual environments as the way to generate them, because the use of web environments promotes the ability and attitude that is suitable for strengthening essential skills in the XXI century. From the systematization of normative documents of Higher Medical Education in Cuba for undergraduate, difficulties are detected in the development of actions during the teaching-learning process from the curriculum in the development of informational competences of human resources who are trained in Health Technology careers at the University of Medical Sciences of Havana, together with the disuse of activities to develop informational competences through the use of ICT. That is why the author proposed to implement a methodological strategy for the use of ICT in the development of informational competences in students of the Faculty of Health Technology of the University of Medical Sciences of Havana. The methodological strategy was validated by experts, students according to a satisfaction survey, as well as by the results during academic performance and from diagnostic instruments at the beginning and end of the implementation.

Key words: ICT, ALFIN, information competencies, methodological strategy, information management.

Table of Contents

INTRODUCTION

Information and communication technologies (ICTs) are currently an important working tool for the dynamization of the scientific research process at all levels. The efficient use of these technologies contributes favorably to a higher degree of technological professionalization of professionals in the process of permanent training, which allows them to face a research according to the advances of society in the present century . [1, 2].

Interest in the study of ICTs is increasing in the different disciplinary fields in which it has repercussions, including the educational field, recognizing the impact it has on education. As time goes by, new technologies and innovations emerge, which is why it is relevant to involve ICT in the teaching and learning process in order to offer a quality and updated education [3]. [3].

In the information society, as it could not be otherwise, the new technologies for accessing, processing and transmitting information, the new forms of communication determine that a large part of the contents and competencies of the basic training required today are directly related to ICT and the media, as reflected in expressions such as computer literacy, audiovisual, multimedia, digital, media, information literacy, all of them related to each other and called to converge . [4].

It is necessary to analyze the definition of competence, which is considered as the mobilization of knowledge, ability, attitude and value that a person shows when acting effectively in the face of various problems based on his or her own characteristics and experiences. Therefore, it refers to a group of knowledge, procedures and attitudes that are combined, in a coordinated and integrated way, in the sense that the person must know how to do and know how to be for professional development [5, 6].

In the knowledge society that humanity is living in, information plays a key role and it is important to acquire information competencies and/or skills in order to effectively access the largest amount of information resources, which will be part of the new knowledge. Therefore, educational institutions cannot remain oblivious to this reality and must ensure that students graduate with information competencies (IC), basic skills to be better professionals and citizens, able to interact and manage the exponential growth of information in a timely manner. [7-9].

At present, digital competencies promote knowledge societies, students and teachers should understand their presence in the various virtual environments as a way to generate them, because the use of web environments promotes the ability and attitude that is suitable for strengthening essential skills in the XXI century. [5, 10-12].

From the epistemological point of view, these transversal competences have an interdisciplinary, multidisciplinary and transdisciplinary character, as they enter into a study that is complex in nature. [1].

Since the end of the 20th century, Higher Education has experienced a progressive shift from the traditional model based on the teaching process to an alternative model based on learning in which students are the protagonists. This new model has been favored by the accelerated development of ICTs and their application in the field of education. The use of these technologies in the educational context has facilitated the development in students of the competencies to self-direct their learning, a process in which the teacher assumes the role of facilitator and guide [13].

Several countries have now proposed to modify their university organic laws, proposing new structures for undergraduate and graduate education in their degree programs. In these institutions, the new curricula for undergraduate degrees incorporate, in addition to subject knowledge, different transversal competencies, among which the use of computer tools and skills in information search, analysis and management stand out [1, 14].

For this reason, ICT are no longer just technological tools in education, but become one of the basic competencies to be developed in the teaching-learning process [11, 15]. [11, 15].

For some years now, Cuba has been going through a process that has been defined as the informatization of society: one of the three pillars that support government management. On this path, Cuba is assuming new precepts that lead it towards digital transformation: a new moment in which digital technologies are integrated in all areas of society, where people are at the center of the process. [16].

In the health sector, the computerization process is one of the key elements of the Strategic Informatization Program of the Ministry of Public Health (MINSAP), the governing body of the National Health System (SNS). This program is implemented in stages in health processes, covering all institutions belonging to the sector (health care, teaching, research and business). [17, 18].

The objective of this program is to increase the quality and optimize services to the population through the impact of the use of ICTs. To achieve this goal, work is carried out in an integrated and systematic manner on three fundamental principles: infrastructure, IT solutions, and human resources training and capacity building. [17].

In the context of underdeveloped countries, health professionals must use ICT to develop information literacy training, be able to identify what information they need to locate, where to find it, how to obtain it, how to analyze it and evaluate it, and then be able to communicate it. [19].

Information literacy in the SNS has its antecedents in the activities of User Education and Bibliographic Instruction that were carried out at the National Center for Medical Sciences Information/Infomed (National Coordinating Body of the Network of Scientific and Technical Information Libraries), the National Medical Library and the various libraries that make up the National System of Scientific and Technical Health Information, long before the 1990s. [20].

From the systematization of normative documents of Higher Medical Education in Cuba for the undergraduate level, difficulties are detected in the development of actions during the teaching-learning process from the curriculum in the development of informational skills of human resources who are trained in Health Technology careers at the University of Medical Sciences of Havana. [19]The study was based on the disuse of activities to develop informational competencies through the use of ICTs.

During the observation carried out in the Faculty of Health Technology of the University of Medical Sciences of Havana, it was detected that the medical library was not able to provide all its services due to the lack of specialized human resources during the year 2022, together with the damages caused to the teaching infrastructure by Hurricane Ian, which damaged part of the classrooms and caused the use of the library as a classroom. During this time, there has been a marked disuse of the ICTs available for the development of students' information competencies.

On the other hand, the Federation of University Students (FEU) held its tenth congress last year. In its session at the faculty level, the students, except for those of the Health Information Systems (HIS) career, issued the following statements:

- There is a lack of information search skills.
- It is necessary to receive the services of the faculty medical library.
- Need for training on access and how to interact in the virtual classroom.

With this background and the author's experience as main professor of the subject Information Competencies in the Health Information Systems career of the Faculty of Health Technology of the University of Medical Sciences of Havana, as a teacher of the mentioned career for more than 13 years since its predecessor in the C and D study plans, being the author of the programs of several subjects and in the exercise of the profession as a graduate of the same, makes it possible to identify the problematic situation that justifies the research: the students of the Faculty of Health Technology of the University of Medical Sciences of Havana, present insufficiencies in the development of IQ during their undergraduate training.

After evaluating the above, a clear contradiction is established between the model of competent information professional demanded by society today and the professional who graduates from university education without developing information competencies. Considering the situation described above, the following theoretical design of the research has been defined:

Research problem: How to contribute to the development of informational competences in students of the Faculty of Health Technology of the University of Medical Sciences of Havana with the use of ICT?

Object of study: Process of development of informational competencies in university students.

Field of action: Development of informational competencies in students of the Faculty of Health Technology of the University of Medical Sciences of Havana with the use of ICT.

Objective System:

General objective: To implement a methodological strategy for the development of informational competencies in students of the Faculty of Health Technology of the University of Medical Sciences of Havana with the use of ICT.

Specific objectives:

1. To characterize the state of the art in the implementation of methodological strategies for the development of informational competencies in higher education through the use of ICTs.
2. To implement the methodological strategy for the development of informational competencies for students of the Faculty of Health Technology of the University of Medical Sciences of Havana with the use of ICT.
3. Validate the methodological strategy based on the criteria of experts and users.

In order to solve the scientific problem and meet the objective, four **scientific questions** with their corresponding tasks are planned, as shown below:

1. What theoretical references support the implementation of methodological strategies for the development of information competencies in higher education through the use of ICTs?

2. What is the status of the development of informational competencies in students of the Faculty of Health Technology of the University of Medical Sciences of Havana?

3. What elements should the methodological strategy for the development of informational competencies with the use of ICT for students of the Faculty of Health Technology of the University of Medical Sciences of Havana have?

4. What results are obtained by implementing the methodological strategy for the development of informational competencies with the use of ICT for students of the Faculty of Health Technology of the University of Medical Sciences of Havana?

The use of the following scientific research methods is highlighted in the research:

Theoretical methods:

- The **analytical-synthetic** for the decomposition of the research problem into elements that allow its individualized analysis in order to discover the general characteristics that can be applied in the proposed methodological strategy.
- The **inductive-deductive method** allowed the passage from particular to general knowledge, by reflecting the coinciding elements in the elements studied and establishing the relationships that these have with each other in the conformation of the substantive elements of the methodological strategy for the development of informational competencies, which facilitated the conception of the proposal.
- The **historical-logical analysis method** for the critical analysis of research associated with the use of ICTs in the development of information competencies, with the objective of establishing a starting point and comparison with the expected results.
- The **documentary analysis** made it possible to frame the process of development of information competencies in the undergraduate program, by systematizing works and outstanding authors on the subject under study.
- **Systematization** was used in the research to learn about the criteria of authors related to the object of research. The coincidence of the different approaches to the use of ICTs in higher education and the development of informational competencies was determined.
- The **modeling** made it possible to elaborate the model of the methodological strategy for the use of ICTs in the development of information competencies by

discovering and studying the existing knowledge on the subject of the respondents and establishing the dialectical relationships of the elements contained in it.

- The **functional structural systemic** approach allowed the identification in the model of the methodological strategy of the interrelationships between the elements necessary for the development of informational competencies through the use of ICTs.

Empirical methods:

- **Observation** was used to assess the main inadequacies that justify the research problem, during the observation of the academic performance of the surveyed students and the theoretical feasibility of the proposed methodological strategy.
- The **survey** to obtain the diagnosis on the need to develop informational competencies with the use of ICT in students, to evaluate the level of satisfaction with the implemented methodological strategy and to know the level of acquisition of competencies after the use of the strategy. The diagnostic instrument and the satisfaction survey were also applied to the experts for the validation of the proposed methodological strategy.

Statistical methods:

Descriptive and inferential statistical methods and techniques were used. Among the descriptive methods, absolute and relative measures were used for qualitative variables (absolute frequencies) and quantitative variables (point arithmetic mean, median, mode and confidence interval). Among the inferential statistical methods, the Mann-Whitney U test (for two independent samples) and the Kruskal-Wallis test (for more than two independent samples) were used. A significance level of five percent was used for both.

Methodological triangulation was applied to collect information, contrast the results, analyze coincidences and differences, which make it possible to assess the change in the development of informational competencies from the academic results achieved and obtain the inventory of problems, as well as the potentialities that characterize the object.

The population defined for the research was the 1912 students who constituted the enrollment of the course 2022, from which a non-probabilistic sample was selected at the discretion of the researcher of 29 students who constituted the enrollment of the fourth year of the regular daytime course of the Health Information Systems course, since it is the only course that receives the informative competences subject in the curriculum. The sample was studied in two conglomerates formed by the two groups taught according to the official enrollment.

For the expert judgment, a non-probabilistic sample of five specialists with experience in the use of ICT in the educational teaching process and information competencies was selected.

Main research contributions.

Contribution to the theory:

- Operational definition of the process of development of informational competences in students of the Faculty of Health Technology of the University of Medical Sciences of Havana.

Practical contributions:

- Methodological strategy for the use of ICT in the development of informational skills in students of the Faculty of Health Technology of the UCM-H.

Proposal validation

The methodological strategy was validated through the criteria of experts and users.

The proposed methodological strategy, the diagnostic questionnaire and the satisfaction survey were evaluated **by experts**. All the instruments were validated by five specialists. The specialists were asked to participate anonymously, having previously signed the informed consent form, and in addition to being considered experts, they had to meet the requirement of being professors linked to the area of knowledge investigated.

By the **users' criterion**, the methodological strategy was evaluated based on the level of satisfaction and by means of the academic results achieved in the subject during the quasi-experiment.

We considered the voluntary participation of the students anonymously, for which we established as inclusion criteria that they were students of the Health Information Systems career of the selected groups, excluding the rest of the students who did not meet the aforementioned criteria and those who of their own free will decided not to remain in the research. They signed the informed consent form.

Structure of the work

The **structure of the paper** consisted of: Introduction, three chapters, Conclusions, Recommendations, and Bibliographical references. Figures and tables were included to facilitate the understanding of the document. The main elements addressed in the three proposed chapters are described below:

In **Chapter 1. Theoretical references of the process of developing informational competencies with the use of information and communication technologies**: a bibliographical review is made on the use of ICT in higher education, the role of ICT in the development of informational competencies and methodological strategies for the use of ICT in the process of developing informational competencies.

In **Chapter 2. Methodological strategy for the use of ICT in the development of informational competences:** the conception of the methodological strategy for the use of ICT in the development of informational competences in the students of the Faculty of Health Technology of the University of Medical Sciences of Havana is described. The theoretical foundations that support the methodological strategy are analyzed. Likewise, the objectives are defined and the actions to be carried out in each activity of the proposed methodological strategy are presented.

Chapter 3. Implementation and assessment of results: presents the implementation process of the designed methodological strategy, including the initial diagnosis and the assessment of the results based on the validation through the criteria of experts and users.

CHAPTER 1: THEORETICAL REFERENCES OF THE PROCESS OF DEVELOPING INFORMATIONAL COMPETENCIES WITH THE USE OF INFORMATION AND COMMUNICATION TECHNOLOGIES

Chapter I. Theoretical references of the process of developing informational competencies with the use of information and communication technologies.

Introduction to the chapter.

The chapter describes the theoretical references that support the methodological strategy for the development of informational competencies with the use of ICTs. It describes the types and structure of competencies, the definition and classification, according to the trend, and the processes implemented for the development of informational competencies in human resources in Medical Sciences.

The main methodologies, strategies and models of training and development of informational competences and the relationship between ICT, their use in higher education and their role in the development of informational competences are systematized. The implementation of a methodological strategy for the use of ICT in the development of informational competences in the students of the Faculty of Health Technology of the University of Medical Sciences of Havana is based.

The process of developing information competencies with the use of information and communication technologies is based on four theoretical cores: process, development, information competencies and information and communication technologies.

1.1.Process

The Dictionary of the Royal Spanish Academy [21] presents several definitions of process, of which the author assumes the following:

1. n. The action of going forward.

2. m. The course of time.

3. m. Set of successive phases of a natural phenomenon or of an artificial operation.

Maldonado [22] states that a process can be defined as a set of interrelated activities that, from one or more inputs of materials or information, give rise to one or more value-added outputs of materials or information. Processes must be properly managed using different process management tools. It also refers to a set of actions and tasks that are performed sequentially, and that together provide added value to customers.

He also points out that the incorporation of new information technologies has made it possible to redefine processes, achieving degrees of effectiveness and efficiency that were unimaginable a few years ago. Likewise, he assumes it as the set of interrelated resources and activities that transform input elements into output elements. Resources may include personnel, finances, facilities, equipment, techniques and methods.

The ISO-9000 series of international standards [23] (quality management systems) defines a process as "a set of mutually related or interacting activities that transform inputs into outputs".

The author, based on the above definitions, assumes for the research the one set forth in the ISO-9000 standards.

1.2. Development

The Dictionary of the Royal Spanish Academy [21] refers, among other meanings, that development is the action and effect of developing or developing, understanding development as the following definitions, according to the objective of this research:

1. To increase or reinforce something of a physical, intellectual or moral order.

2. To state an issue or topic in an orderly and comprehensive manner.

3. To perform or carry out something. He developed an important work.

4. Said of a human community: To progress or grow, especially in the economic, social sphere.

Development is a historical concept, which means that it does not have a single definition, but has evolved according to the dominant thinking and values of society [24].

The concept of development is related to the idea of the future that each society proposes as a goal for the human collective. Development must be understood as a future category. When we establish the priorities of what we understand by development, in the final analysis, we are simply stating our vision of what we want in the future. [24].

One of the most controversial concepts is that of development (referring to the development of a country). There is no consensus in the literature, so that it is possible to find several definitions, in some cases incompatible [25].

Based on the above systematization, the author assumes for the research the first definition issued by the Dictionary of the Royal Spanish Academy, which refers to increasing or reinforcing something of a physical, intellectual or moral order.

1.3. Information Competencies

1.3.1. Competencies. Definition. Types and structure.

The term competence comes from the Latin *competentia*, from the 15th century meaning to concern, belong to, correspond to, giving rise to the noun competence with the meaning of "that which corresponds to a person to do with responsibility and suitability" and the adjective competent with the meaning apt or adequate.

It is defined by emphasizing various aspects within the framework of the establishment of innovative methodologies to evaluate learning and the quality of education, as a change from methodologies based on memorization and mechanical repetition of data to recognize cognitive processes -perception, attention, comprehension, intelligence and language- and cognitive capacities -interpretation, argumentation and proposition-, in order to improve the evaluation of learning, taking into account approaches based on know-how in context. Thus, the concept of competencies is incorporated into formal education from the field of language, from linguistic competence and communicative competence [26].

According to Gardner's theory of multiple intelligences, all human beings possess to a greater or lesser extent eight types of intelligence that may or may not manifest themselves depending on different cultural and environmental factors: linguistic, naturalistic, musical, intrapersonal, interpersonal, logical-mathematical, visuospatial and bodily-kinesthetic. Taking into account this multiplicity, competencies could be conceptualized as Tobón states (definition assumed by the author for the research):

"Integral processes of action between activities and problems of personal life, the community, society, the ecological environment, the work-professional context, science, organizations, art and recreation, contributing to the construction and transformation of reality, for which the knowledge of being (self-motivation, initiative, values and collaborative work with others) is integrated with the knowledge of knowing (conceptualizing, interpreting, and arguing) and knowing how to do (applying procedures and strategies), taking into account the specific challenges of the environment, personal growth needs and personal growth processes, values and collaborative work with others) with knowing how to know (conceptualize, interpret, and argue) and knowing how to do (apply procedures and strategies), taking into account the specific challenges of the environment, personal growth needs and processes of uncertainty, with a spirit of challenge, suitability and ethical commitment." [26].

The Directorate General for Education and Culture of the European Commission, in the Culture Programme 2007-13 [27]27], considers that the term "competence" refers to a combination of skills, knowledge, aptitudes and attitudes, and to the inclusion of the willingness to learn, in addition to knowing how:

"Key competencies represent a multifunctional and transferable package of knowledge, skills and attitudes that all individuals need for personal fulfillment and development, inclusion and employment."

In the educational field, competencies are considered to be integral actions that arise from an education oriented to the development of the different potentialities of the subject, considering his or her context and the different educational scenarios, as well as their multidimensionality. They can be classified as specific and basic-generic. [26]:

- Specific competencies: These are those specific to a certain occupation or profession, therefore, they have a high degree of specialization, as well as specific educational processes (technical programs, job training and higher education).
- Basic-generic competencies: Also known as cross-cutting competencies, they are essential for personal fulfillment, they enable and qualify for successful integration into professional, labor and social life, and can be trained in basic, middle and higher education.

Competencies "are acquired through systematic teaching and learning processes in the family, society and educational institutions". These were systematized by the CIFE Institute based on international projects, among them: Scans 1992, Tuning 2005 and DeSeCo 2005. [26]. The following essential basic-generic competencies are identified:

1) Self-management of training
2) Oral and written communication
3) Oral and written communication in a second language
4) Teamwork and leadership
5) Information and knowledge management
6) Math-based problem solving
7) Natural science-based problem solving
8) Entrepreneurship
9) Research
10) Quality management.

Competencies are currently defined and classified according to their tendency to depend on the actions of professionals, in relation to the attitudes, skills and values they maintain in their modes of action . [28].

They constitute the objective basis necessary to integrate both the processes developed by each individual and these at work, social life, the place and historical period in which professional life is developed, the interrelation of the teaching and care process in which they work, which will respond to the needs of society and could be considered to support the balance between professionals with academic centers that train human resources. [28].

1.3.2. Information competencies. Definitions and models.

In information and knowledge management skills, with the technological advances and the amount of information volumes that are permanently generated and disseminated, it is essential to consider the criteria in the information search strategy in its selection, classification, retrieval, analysis and use, taking into account intellectual property and the diversity of sources. [26, 29-32].

The above depends on several factors, among them the informational skills or competencies required by an individual, and to a great extent it is the responsibility of educational institutions to contribute to their training by strengthening learning and research through skills in the use, management and communication of information. Therefore, it is important to have spaces that contribute to the processes of integral formation of the educational community to generate processes of knowledge acquisition on information skills that favor the transformation of information into new knowledge. [26, 33-35].

The American Association of School defines information competency as follows. [36] as the "ability to recognize a need for information and the ability to identify, locate, evaluate, organize, communicate, and use information effectively for both problem solving and lifelong learning." [27].

Information literacy, according to the Joint Commission of the Conference of Rectors of Spanish Universities (CRUE-TIC) and the University Library Network (REBIUN), is "the set of knowledge, skills, dispositions and behaviors that enable individuals to recognize when they need information, where to locate it, how to assess its suitability and how to use it appropriately according to the problem they face." [37].

Quindemil Torrijo EM [38] assumes that information competencies are acquired through information literacy and are defined as the set of abilities, knowledge, skills, attitudes and values to define an information need, search, find, select, evaluate, use and communicate information effectively, with an ethical, reflective and critical sense. This definition of informational competencies is the one assumed by the author for the research.

González García, in his doctoral thesis, addresses the competence in Information Management as one of the five research competencies with an interdisciplinary approach to health technologies, defining them as the development of skills in the search for and processing of information with the use of new technologies, for the efficient and optimal use of resources. Aimed at locating information sources and processing them, as well as organizing the bibliography using the standards established in each case. [39].

Informational competencies infer aspects of each individual, from the emotional to the cognitive and attitudinal, associated with skills in the use of technologies, access to networks in the search, information management, as well as the need for autonomous learning; at the same time, they involve others when interacting in a context; being dynamic and changeable as one progresses as a social being.

Based on the ALFIN proposals and standards, models have emerged, developed by the ACRL/ ALA 2000 (Developed by the Association of College and Research Libraries), in the United States, the ANZIIL, in Australia and New Zealand. [19, 40-42]some of which can be implemented, coincide in the methodology and in the mastery of competencies to determine, access, evaluate, use and understand many of the problems related to the use of information, as well as to use it ethically and lawfully [33-35].

The models to be applied in an ALFIN program should have a multidisciplinary approach that allows teaching and learning, stimulates critical thinking, allows the interrelation between students, teachers and librarians, to relate the daily activities with the subjects included in the curriculum. [19, 41, 43].

The author agrees with the review by Zelada,[19] who systematized some of the theoretical models for teaching IC available in the literature consulted. On the basis of the systematization carried out, Zelada [19] classifies them according to the processes at which they are aimed. Some of the models constitute tools for the organization of the processes of: search, evaluation, processing, and dissemination or communication of information [19, 27, 44, 45].

The most widespread and systematized models are: Gavilan Model and Gavilan 2.0 Model, OSLA Model, Stripling Pitts Model, Kuhlthau Model or Information Seeking Process (ISP), Marland and Irving Model, James Herring's PLUS Model, SCONUL Model of project-based learning, BRUCE Model, Benito Morales' documentary education model.

Finally, the Big6 Model is discussed [19, 44, 46] developed by Mike Eisenberg and Bob Berkowitz. It is a systematic process of information problem solving supported by critical thinking. It could also be defined as the six skill areas necessary for effective and efficient information problem solving (specific and strategic points that help meet information needs) or as a complete curriculum of library use and information management skills.

1.3.3. Informational competencies in health professionals.

The circumscription of information competencies in higher education brings with it recourse to the different norms that, at the international level, declare the evaluative standards that determine when a student is or is not competent in information. These standards appeared in the year 2000 by the Association of College and Research Libraries (ACRL/ALA) and, indistinctly, organizations of the profession in different regions have included other considerations, indicators and objectives, declaring in them as common denominator the linking of teachers and librarians to develop ALFIN proposals that lead to the formation of a competent information professional. [19, 38].

The core competencies, contextualized and adapted to the conditions of the National Health System in Cuba, become an indispensable requirement to ensure that professionals in the sector incorporate knowledge, skills and attitudes for the proper management of scientific information. The elements described in each competency define the contents of the teaching-learning process of these competencies and specify "the level of competencies for a person to acquire the skills that make him/her information literate at a certain evolutionary stage" [47, 48] [47, 48]. [47, 48].

These standards encourage "the individual to become aware of his or her knowledge, which includes "know-how", "know-how" and "know-how" that allows him or her to put into practice his or her potential to transfer and learn throughout his or her life" [47, 49] [47, 49]. [47, 49].

The Core Competencies define that a worker in the context of health sciences is competent in information management if he/she has the ability to. [47, 50, 51]:

Determine the Information Need.

2. Properly locate and access the information you need.

3. Assess information for authenticity, correctness, value and bias.

4. Organize information and use it effectively.

5. Expand, restructure or create new knowledge by integrating previous knowledge with the knowledge you have acquired.

6. Recognize ethics and responsibility in the use of information.

7. Recommend and/or undertake appropriate actions based on the analysis of the information.

Zelada [19] in his research, from a dialectical materialist approach, decides to build a model for his research, which relates from the teacher's job, his tasks and functions to develop their modes of action, from the context of CI.

From the analysis presented by Zelada [19, 50, 51] allowed him to identify for the research four ICs to achieve its development in the teachers of the University of Medical Sciences of Havana.

1. Competence in motivation for learning IQs

2. Competent performance in the evaluation of information

3. Information acquisition and processing competence

4. Competence in communication and dissemination of information

1.3.4. Informational competencies for Health Technology students.

According to Zelada [19]the systematization of normative documents on medical education shows the absence of actions to acquire IC during the teaching-learning process, from undergraduate studies in medical science professionals, who will be trained in graduate studies as teachers or tutors in the performance of professional activities in the teaching-care area, with the exception of the Bachelor's degree in SIS.

In the structure of the study plan of the SIS career in curriculum D, the core curriculum includes the main integrating discipline CI and collaborative work environments in network, technical discipline to deal with Scientific Information and Medical Librarianship, thus achieving a graduate with the required CI.

The conception of the subject for this curriculum focuses on the theoretical and practical aspects of information literacy as well as the formation of the information competencies established by Fernandez [20] for health professionals. Likewise, it assumes the competencies for teachers proposed by Zelada [19]It prepares students as teachers by assigning them the role of teachers in the practical activity in order to design courses in a virtual teaching-learning environment using the Moodle platform from the theoretical aspects received.

Based on the author's experience as a teacher of the subject and on the knowledge acquired in provincial and national courses on the subject, it is considered necessary to analyze the training in informational competences in Health Technology students in general, framed in the post-pandemic context of COVID-19, where the use of virtual spaces in the teaching process played a determining role in the continuity of teaching in the country. For this reason, the proposal assumes the use of ICT for the development of informational competencies.

The author assumes the seven core informational competencies established by Fernandez [20] for health professionals mentioned in the previous section and adjusts them to the undergraduate environment in university education and to the current situation of Cuban society.

1.4. Information and Communications Technologies.

1.4.1. Definitions.

According to Law 1341 of Colombia [52] ICTs are the set of resources, tools, equipment, computer programs, applications, networks and media that allow the compilation, processing, storage and transmission of information such as voice, data, text, video and images.

The National Medical Library of Cuba [53] states that information and communication technologies (ICT) are all those tools and programs that process, manage, transmit and share information by means of technological supports. Computers, the Internet and telecommunications are the most widespread ICTs, although their growth and evolution are causing more and more models to emerge.

On the other hand, Belloch [54] states that ICTs are the set of technologies that allow access, production, processing and communication of information presented in different codes (text, image, sound,...).

Other definitions refer to the fact that, in general terms, ICTs are the set of technological tools and solutions that make it possible to streamline, organize and process the information and communications of people, companies and organizations in favor of efficiency and agility. [55].

It can also be said to be the practices and knowledge connected to the consumption and transmission of information developed and enhanced after the digital transformation [55].

The Latin University of Costa Rica [56] defines ICT as the resources and tools used for the process, administration and distribution of information through technological elements, such as: computers, telephones, televisions, etc.

Cobo [57] citing Fernandez [58] states that ICTs are collectively defined as innovations in microelectronics, computing (hardware and software), telecommunications and optoelectronics - microprocessors, semiconductors, fiber optics - that allow the processing and accumulation of enormous amounts of information, as well as a rapid distribution of information through communication networks.

1.4.2. Information and communication technologies in the training of human resources.

Since the end of the 20th century, Higher Education has experienced a progressive shift from the traditional model based on the teaching process to an alternative model based on learning in which students are the protagonists. This new model has been favored by the accelerated development of ICT and its application in the field of education. [6].

The use of ICTs in the educational context has facilitated the development in students of the competencies for self-directed learning. In this process, the teacher assumes the role of facilitator and guide, while the leading role corresponds to the students. [6].

The training of human resources is fundamentally centered on two stages: general education, which extends from early childhood to the pre-university level, and university education. The latter has two fundamental stages: undergraduate and postgraduate.

It is in general education where the basic competencies of the human being should be formed and developed, since they are the ones that will accompany him/her throughout life and contribute to his/her intellectual development in the course of his/her education. In the case of specific competencies, these are formed in undergraduate education according to the profession, which are consolidated and expanded in postgraduate education.

In several countries, as is the case of Cuba, polytechnic education is included within the general education, so that a significant number of individuals train and develop the specific competencies of the profession in the very education in which their basic competencies are formed, to later expand and consolidate them in the continuation of university studies or in the practice of the profession.

ICTs play a fundamental role in this process. The process of computerization that today's society is undergoing has had an impact not only on work environments but also on education. In this field, educational technology emerges, with two fundamental aspects. [59]:

- Educational software, audiovisual materials or mobile applications to teach different subjects.
- A new pedagogical model is also an example of educational technology, since it involves a series of teaching techniques and procedures. Concepts such as systems theory are used. At present, Information and Communication Technologies -ICT's- have also been incorporated into educational technology through the Internet, computers and mobile telephony, among other areas.

Educational technology has reshaped the way of teaching, as it keeps the teachers in the area connected to the global world in order to give the most knowledge and streamline the learning process, using all the tools that technology provides us with [59].

Technology is influencing the world of education in at least two ways: one related to pedagogical, administrative and school management interests; and the other to changes in the skills and competencies required to carry out an education in tune with the proposed objectives [59]. [59].

Thus, education has been and is being strongly influenced by the insertion of ICT in schools, which can be seen, for example in [59].

- Resource optimization.
- The improvement of teaching and learning processes.
- An education aimed at "learning to learn".
- Generate training in relation to new sources of information.
- Improve the harmony between school and society.

1.4.3. Information and communication technologies in the formation of informational competencies.

As previously mentioned by the author, IQs are considered basic - generic, however, they have a particularity, at the same time they are specific competencies.

As basic - generic competencies, they are considered to be an indispensable element in the daily life of any human being in the information and communications era, where ICTs play a determining role in the entire information management cycle.

From the point of view of specific competence, it is considered as such because it is a distinctive element of information professionals, mainly in the library field. It is for this reason that the training of IC has been a function historically assigned to the library field worldwide, a trend that even today, despite being a widely addressed issue and of imperative need to transform, continues to exert a strong influence on the training process.

In analyzing the process of formation of the ICs, it is essential to start from user education, a service provided by libraries that was responsible for training people in the skills needed to search for the necessary information and create competencies in them within the scope of institutions of this type, whether public, educational, institutional or private.

The emergence and rapid development of ICTs led to a paradigm shift in the information management process. The digitization of information has conditioned an obsolescence of printed literature to encourage greater consumption of information through various digital platforms, to the point of currently having digital libraries, just to mention one of the digital information resources.

1.5. Process of development of information competencies with the use of ICTs.

Based on the systematization carried out after the analysis and evaluation of the scientific literature consulted on the topic of study, the following generalities can be determined in the process of developing informational competencies with the use of ICTs:

- Some authors and regions use the term information literacy and others, as a synonym, information competencies.
- It is assumed in today's society that ICTs are an intrinsic part of the process of training and development of information competencies.
- Information competencies continue to be mostly seen as specific to information professionals and are not promoted as basic-generic for all people.
- The training and development of information competencies in Cuba is assumed through training courses, mainly for postgraduate students.
- There is a tendency to strengthen the formative processes of information competencies at the undergraduate level, with concrete actions in some universities based on elective courses, as well as the establishment of theoretical-methodological conceptions and didactic strategies for their formation.

The author, based on the evaluation of the literature and his own experience, states that information competencies are the result of information literacy, assuming the concept that information competencies are acquired through the process of information literacy, in which not only the development of information skills is conceived, but the formation of values related to the process of information management. [60-63].

At the same time, it was not found a theoretical conceptualization of the process of development of informational competences with the use of ICT, so the author, for the research, defines operationally the process of development of informational competences with the use of ICT in students of the Faculty of Health Technology of the UCM-H as the:

[...] a set of methodologically organized and interrelated actions to develop informational competencies during undergraduate studies, based on knowledge, the development of skills that allow an adequate professional performance and the values that should characterize them in relation to information, allowing an effective management of information and knowledge with the use of ICT.

Conclusions of the chapter

The theoretical framework that supports the development of IQ through the use of ICTs was described. The main methodologies, strategies and models of training and development of information competencies and the use of ICT in higher education were systematized, as well as the role of ICT in the development of information competencies. An operational definition of the process of development of informational competences with the use of ICTs in students of the Faculty of Health Technology of the University of Medical Sciences of Havana was established.

CHAPTER 2: METHODOLOGICAL STRATEGY FOR THE DEVELOPMENT OF INFORMATIONAL COMPETENCIES WITH THE USE OF INFORMATION AND COMMUNICATION TECHNOLOGIES

Chapter II. Methodological strategy for the development of informational competencies with the use of information and communication technologies.

Introduction to the chapter

This chapter describes the theoretical references that support the implementation of the proposed methodological strategy. The methodological strategy is operationally defined with the use of information and communication technologies for the formation of informational competences in the students of the Faculty of Health Technology of the University of Medical Sciences of Havana, which is described from the elements that integrate it. The objectives, theoretical foundations and competencies that are present in the strategy are described, as well as the stages, phases and methodological actions that integrate it.

2.1. Theoretical references that support the implementation of the methodological strategy.

2.1.1. The development of information competencies in undergraduate education

Internationally, there are examples of the inclusion of information literacy training from the undergraduate level. Such is the case of the Library of the Law School of the Universidad UDELAR, in Montevideo, where Chávez and González [64] present a report that states that, together with the progress in the new curriculum, it is in a dynamic of constant change due to the new needs and behaviors of users due to the adoption of new learning models. The librarian has ceased to be a mere intermediary of information to fulfill formative functions being part of the collaborative learning that is imposed.

They also state that the changes that have occurred in the academic environment have forced libraries, and especially the reference service, not only to have the appropriate tools, but also, in the first instance, to be trained in their information skills in order to develop the information competencies necessary for users to acquire and use information in a critical and creative way, and to continue in an autonomous process of constant training.

The author considers it important to analyze that in Cuba the scenario for the development of informational competencies is still considered the postgraduate activity. This is in contradiction with the classification of competencies expressed by Hernandez

[26]who states that informational competencies are basic-generic, therefore, they should be developed in parallel with the intellectual development of the individual from an early age.

This statement is also supported by Machado and Montes de Oca [65]65], who, based on the systematization of theory and practice, offer criteria on the essential requirements for designing competency-based curricula from the perspective of the historical-cultural approach, while confirming that curriculum design requires a high degree of specialization, an eye to the future, creativity and innovation, development of research competencies, humanity, experience and a sense of belonging to the context in which future graduates will carry out their professional work.

Following this idea, the author reaffirms that the curricula of undergraduate education in the country still contemplate training by objectives, not by competencies, which, in the case of Health Technology careers, are concentrated in Work Education. However, in the case of CI, it should be noted that they do not appear in the curricula of the aforementioned university careers, except for the Health Information Systems career, whose curriculum includes CI training as a subject, and therefore it is taught in a curricular manner.

For undergraduate education, meanwhile, steps have been taken in terms of training and development of IC through courses and information literacy programs, among other actions. Among them, the following authors can be mentioned.

Valverde and Rosales [66] proposed a program for the formation of informational competencies in Stomatology undergraduate students, as a proposal for an undergraduate elective course, aimed at developing informational competencies for the solution of teaching problems and research tasks. They carried out a pedagogical research in which the core competences 1 and 2 defined in the Norms of informational competences of the National System of Information in Health Sciences in Cuba were reviewed and adapted, and the results of the diagnoses of the research training in the Stomatology career and of the level of knowledge of the first year students of the same career were taken into account.

Suarez [67] at the Universidad de las Ciencias Informáticas presented a theoretical-methodological conception for information literacy in the preparation for employment of graduates who are linked to teaching in the Computer Science Engineering career at the UCI. Similarly, at the university itself, Estrada, Fuentes and Simón [68]68], addressed the formation of informational competencies in Bioinformatics from undergraduate studies with the proposal of a didactic model to achieve this objective.

Based on the author's experience, he assumes that IQs today should be trained from early ages, but in his role as a university professor, he assumes the responsibility of promoting their development from the undergraduate level, since they are not trained by the current general education. That is why he proposes to promote the development of IQ from the curriculum from the subject Information Competences and Collaborative Work Environments in Network with the use of ICT. To achieve this objective, the present research proposes to implement a methodological strategy for the use of ICT in the process of developing informational competencies in the students of the Faculty of Health Technology of the UCM-H.

2.1.2. Parameterization of variables

The process of parameterization according to Añorga J. "is the derivation made as a result of the analysis of the object and/or field of study in the research with measurable or observable elements that allow the assessment or issuance of value judgments about the state, level or development of the phenomenon or process under investigation. The purpose of parameterization is to delve deeper into the phenomenon or object under investigation and can serve for: diagnosis, characterization, validation, verification, demonstration and/or ascertainment" [39, 69, 70].

Gonzalez [39] refers that the parameterization allows to determine the variable with which we are going to work in the research, to define dimensions, indicators and the instruments that will allow to deepen in the object and the field, quoting Lazo [71]who at the same time stated that for Artiles et. al. [72]variables are "the quantitative or qualitative characteristics or properties of the phenomenon under study, which acquire different values, magnitudes or intensities, varying with respect to the units of observation".

In determining the variable, González [39] refers to Campistrous L. et al. [73]73], in recognizing as variables those concepts or general qualities, which are used to represent any of the particular states of the aspect of reality to be studied; these states are the values of the variable and, in each particular manifestation, in each specific case, the variable assumes one of these values.

By taking into consideration the above definitions, the author determines that the independent variable is the methodological strategy for the use of ICT and the dependent variable is the process of developing informational competencies in the students of the Faculty of Health Technology at UCM-H.

Independent variable

The independent variable "methodological strategy for the use of ICTs" is made up of three levels (internal, external and contextual), four stages (awareness and diagnosis, planning, implementation and control and, finally, evaluation). At the same time, each stage is subdivided into phases. The integration of the stages and phases allows the development of a number of methodological actions aimed at solving the problems detected, motivated by the change from the current state to the desired one. It implies a planning process in which there is the establishment of sequences of actions oriented towards the end to be achieved; which does not mean a single course of the same, because they are dialectically interrelated in a global plan of the objectives or ends to be pursued and the methodology to achieve them, aspects in which the author coincides with the research carried out by Lorenzo [74].

Dependent variable

The dependent variable is the process of development of informational competencies in the students of the Faculty of Health Technology at UCM-H was defined by the author in Chapter I and is analyzed according to dimensions.

According to González [39]the Diccionario de la Lengua Española [21] states that the term dimension is defined as "the length or extension of an object in a given direction".

In determining the dimensions, the author took into account what was stated by González [39] who refers to Borges [75] on what, in 2001, González and Valcárcel stated. [76]that they are "(...) those features that will facilitate a first division within the concept" that is, the different parts or attributes to be analyzed in an object, process or phenomenon expressed in a concept or simply different directions of analysis".

In this sense, the author defines four dimensions: informational knowledge, informational skills, informational attitudes and informational aptitudes. For a better understanding and interpretation of these, we refer to his arguments.

Dimension 1: informational knowledge, associated with knowing how to know, is based on the ability to conceptualize, interpret and argue about the information required by the student to face any situation in practical life and in his/her professional environment. It expresses the level of knowledge acquired through the contents of the subject on informational competencies.

Dimension 2: informational skills, associated with know-how. It denotes the skills in applying the informational steps, methods, procedures and strategies. It examines how the student executes the necessary skills to consolidate and develop the acquired knowledge to efficiently assume the management of information and knowledge.

Dimension 3: informational attitudes, associated with knowing how to be. It evaluates self-motivation, initiative, values and collaborative work around information and knowledge management. It takes into account the disposition, independence, autonomy, respect and ethics regarding intellectual property, commitment, self-management of learning in correspondence with the advances of ICT, and it also assumes compliance with professional ethics in the different contexts to which they are assigned.

Dimension 4: informational skills, related to knowing how to be. It assumes taking into account the specific challenges of the student in his environment, taking into consideration personal growth needs and uncertainty processes, with a spirit of challenge, suitability and ethical commitment around information.

After the interpretation of the declared dimensions, the indicators of these dimensions are determined, which result in a total of 28, distributed uniformly, seven in each dimension, numbered consecutively according to the number assigned to them.

After operationalizing the variable, a measurement value was assigned to the indicators based on a four-position ordinal scale: [4 (high)], [3 (medium)], [2 (low)], [1 (none)].

2.1.3. Methodological Strategy Models

The use of strategies in the educational field has transformed the ways of working in the classroom because it promotes the integration of innovative pedagogical and didactic tasks focused on the achievement of expected learning in students [77, 78]. [77, 78]. In turn, Suárez, Palacios and Vera [77] summarize that Magallán, Franco and Tobar [79]state that strategies refer to the ability to propose and guide; the strategist programs, organizes and directs the teaching tasks for the achievement of the established purposes. In addition, they comprise a number of cognitive processes that students use to organize the information obtained and thus understand the processes and the different intellectual actions.

Suarez, Palacios and Vera [77] Systematize the research of Aguilar-Gordón. [80] on teaching methodologies and their influence on the inter-learning process in the subject of Spanish allowed identifying shortcomings in the area and proposing alternatives for improvement through a work guide, with active methodological strategies that actively stimulate the students' commitment, which was applied by the teachers, The research proposal was approached in a sequential manner by teachers and was monitored by the directors.

Mero [81] proposes in his research a methodological strategy consisting of four stages, and describes within each stage the activities to be developed. The stages described by him are: design and development of the methodological strategy; implementation and evaluation of the strategy; analysis of results; and, finally, dissemination and socialization of the results.

Suarez [82] proposes in his research a theoretical-methodological conception for information literacy in preparation for employment in the career of Computer Science at the University of Computer Science, within which he conceives a methodological strategy composed of four stages (familiarization and diagnosis, planning, execution and evaluation and feedback), phases and methodological actions.

Valley [83] proposes a structure in which the components of the strategy are the mission, objectives, actions, methods and procedures, resources, those responsible for the actions and the time in which they should be carried out, the forms of implementation and finally the forms of evaluation.

Zelada [19] structured the Curricular Model for the formation of IC in teachers of the University of Medical Sciences of Havana considering the abstraction of practice coupled with the author's experience in work performance, which allowed her modeling in components, phases and stages.

The author, from the systematization of the different models, assumes the one proposed by Valle [83] adjusted to the structures presented by Suárez [67] and Zelada [19]from which he elaborates his own structure that can be seen in item 2.3.1.

2.2. Methodological strategy for the development of information competencies using information and communication technologies.

The model for the methodological strategy for the formation of informational competencies with the use of information and communication technologies is based on the existing contradiction between the professional who is trained in higher education today, using as a case study the students of the Faculty of Health Technology, which lacks training in informational competencies in digital environments and the competent professional in information and knowledge management with the use of ICTs that contemporary society demands. The proposed model can be seen in Figure 1.

Figure 1. Methodological strategy for the development of information competencies with the use of ICTs.

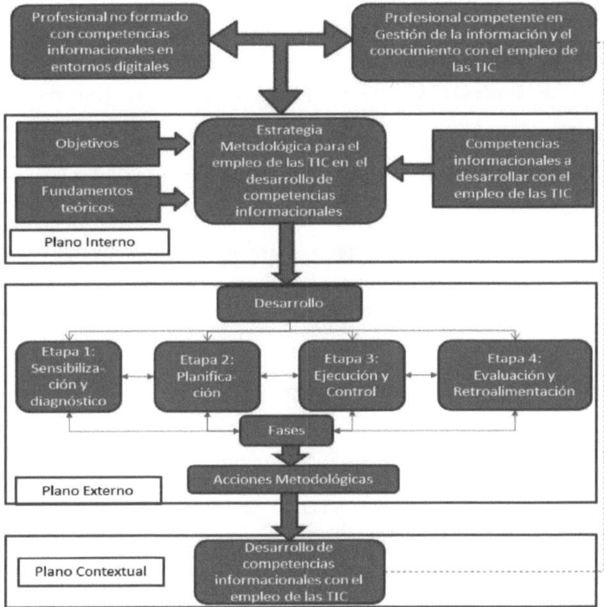

The proposed model is composed of three levels (internal, external and contextual). The internal level establishes the objectives of the methodological strategy, the theoretical foundations that support it, as well as the informational competencies to be developed with the use of ICTs.

The external plan is made up of four stages and several phases, which vary in number depending on the stage; within which the methodological actions to be developed are established, bearing in mind the general objectives of the methodological strategy and the specific objectives of each stage, phase and activity.

The contextual level shows the development achieved from the implementation of the methodological strategy. The results achieved are discussed in chapter III of the research.

2.3. Description of the methodological strategy for the development of informational competencies with the use of information and communication technologies in students of Health Technology at the University of Medical Sciences of Havana.

The methodological strategy, as shown in figure 1 in the previous chapter, is made up of plans, in which stages, phases, as well as methodological elements such as objectives, fundamentals, and methodological actions, among others, converge. The structure of the proposal is shown below.

2.3.1. Internal plane

Objectives of the methodological strategy:

Overall objective

To develop informational competencies in the students of the Faculty of Health Technology of the University of Medical Sciences of Havana with the use of ICT.

Specific objectives:

Strengthen the use of ICTs in the process of developing information competencies.

To develop the seven core competencies defined for health professionals in Cuba from the undergraduate level.

Theoretical foundations that support the methodological strategy:

Philosophical: Marxist-Leninist philosophy, based on its dialectical-materialist method in direct relation to the process of man's formation in interaction with nature and society, through social practice, takes into account the development of the scientific conception of the world.

From the analysis of the pedagogical process in which the influence of various factors is considered, the changes that occur, the experience gained by the students during the curricular training, the correct interpretation between the content of the theory and the objective reality and the establishment of a close relationship with life.

The methodological strategy based on the Marxist-Leninist theory of knowledge is conceived so that, starting from the problems related to the professional profile, the student can determine the need for information, search, analyze and interpret the information, organize it and be able to acquire the knowledge, skills and values necessary to use them when performing his work in any of the different scenarios of professional performance. It considers practice as the beginning and the end of cognitive activity.

It also considers the role of contradictions in the process for the acquisition of knowledge and the need to determine, among others, those that are manifested between the new knowledge, skills and values acquired by students during the training process and intellectual production in the context of health care during on-the-job education at different levels of health care.

Between theoretical knowledge and the ability to apply it in practice during IC training, there is the level of the contents that are the object of study in each research or practical problem of professional work, from the workplace and the real possibilities for their assimilation. This constitutes a driving force to be taken into account in the methodological strategy for the development of IC in FATESA students at the University of Medical Sciences of Havana.

It is based on the position that the student must assume in the constant self-preparation to improve his way of thinking, feeling and acting in order to achieve the highest quality in the evaluations. To solve the academic problems of the students, from the enrichment of their knowledge, skills and values that this path offers. It takes into account the project and the protocolization of IQ training at the different levels of professional performance as a social historical phenomenon that occurs in stages towards higher levels.

Legal: It is specified in all the guiding documents analyzed and used in the research, such as: Agenda 2030; the PCC Guidelines; RM 47/22 Organizational Regulation of the teaching process and of the direction of teaching and methodological work for university careers; the model of the professional in Health Technology careers; RM of the MES on the Model of professional training in Cuba; the Bases of the national plan for economic and social development until 2030: vision of the nation, axes and strategic sectors, among other guiding documents of Cuban medical education.

Psychological: The methodological strategy is based on the psychology that assumes the cultural-historical paradigm developed by Vygotsky. [19, 84] and his followers.

It is based on the conception of the zone of proximal development, in which the diagnosis of each student plays an important role in order to carry out research and professional problem solving at any of the levels of health care where he/she develops education at work, essential for continuity as a permanent process.

It constitutes the basis for perceiving and executing actions aimed at receiving the necessary help and stimulating self-learning to achieve transit to the desired levels.

The strategy considers the systematic exchange among students, based on respectful communication and in which they play an active role in discussing the methodological strategy for the development of IQ in FATESA students at the University of Medical Sciences of Havana.

By exchanging criteria related to the problems identified, reflecting critically on professional problems, as well as the constant interest in the search for solutions to transform reality and acquire knowledge, skills and attitudes.

By taking into account the unity of the affective and the cognitive. The realization of individual and collective tasks contributes to deepen the basic contents to direct the integral development of the personality of the students and the stimulation of the achievements reached.

Sociological: The analysis of principles, theories and models made it possible to identify problems developed in the social relevance of the methodological strategy.

Sociological relevance to informational aspects is a growing demand in society, as information is a social phenomenon and a tool for empowerment, so that any activity related to information must address its social foundations.

The training of students is a priority for the SNS and the University of Medical Sciences, this being its primary social purpose, which will be in correspondence with the quality of the academic performance of students.

Cuban society requires better prepared students to successfully develop their work, in correspondence with the growing progress of the informatization process, which increasingly demands the incorporation of a sociological perspective to the phenomena of information, in accordance with the demands of today's society.

The proposed methodological strategy is an alternative to prepare students from the academic performance, thus raising the level of competence and performance in relation to information, in correspondence with today's society and scientific and technological development, to apply the basic principles of education and help train human resources with quality.

Pedagogical: The proposed methodological strategy is based on Marxist-Leninist and Martian pedagogical conceptions on which Cuban pedagogy is based, with the aim of achieving unity between the instructive, educational and developmental aspects.

It is assumed the need to organize improvement in relation to life, to adapt the methodological strategy to the real conditions of the territory, to the problems related to health education and to the moments of the transformations taking place in the SNS, in order to link the process with the social context.

It assumes the pedagogical foundation and techniques, as it provides mastery of modern methods and procedures in the field of education and teaching, as well as pedagogical influence on the student.

The pedagogical process, in correspondence with pedagogy, concentrates its attention on the study of the activity of the educator and the student. It is the basis on which the theory and methodology are elaborated, as well as the organization and the content, methods, procedures and means are perfected.

The methodological strategy itself favors the development of the research process in a stratified way; it is important to consider the characteristics of all those involved in the process of developing information competencies.

The indispensable relationship between the components responsible for the process, as well as between these and the methodological strategy for the development of IQ in FATESA students of the University of Medical Sciences of Havana is taken into account.

It is considered that the student remains as an active subject, by the constant and conscious improvement when interacting with others, from the construction of knowledge, as a guide of appropriate behaviors.

Based on the experience they will gain and their attitudes, they will guide their personal development and the improvement of their academic performance and pre-professional practice activities from the different scenarios of education at work.

Planned work methods are established, based on the principles of contemporary medical education, where the student, under the guidance of the teacher, develops the teaching-learning process as an active and responsible entity, which will be in correspondence with the academic results achieved.

In the development of CI from the methodological strategy, the laws of pedagogy referred to by Dr. Chávez et al. [19, 85]starting from considering professional improvement and performance as pedagogical processes associated with the social character of man's education in the process of permanent and continuous preparation.

Thus, the proposed methodological strategy considers all the socio-cultural environments surrounding the students of the Faculty of Health Technology of the University of Medical Sciences of Havana, such as the work and personal environment, considering that their performance is developed in the scenarios of education at work.

Didactic: It is essentially contained in the methodological strategy. Every process of development of informational competences has implicit Didactics and is assumed as the science that studies the teaching-learning process aimed at preparing man for life, based on the unity between the instructive, the educational and the developmental, the methodology, the procedures to be used and the relationships between the didactic categories (objectives, contents, methods, teaching means, forms of organization and evaluation). These relationships between the components are highlighted, starting from the ALFIN as a teaching problem, enhancing the guiding role of the objective.

Medical Education: Throughout the process of modeling the methodological strategy, Medical Education is present, so that ICs can be developed. The principles of on-the-job education, permanent and continuing education, teaching-healthcare and research integration, performance improvement and professional and human behavior are expressed.

The methodological strategy is based on the educational theory of Medical Education, which aims at professional and human improvement, as well as the historical-cultural approach, based on the assumption:

- the personalized treatment of the students participating in the training actions, from the characterization of the development of IQ in the students. The informational problems that arise in this development process, expressed in the fulfillment of their curricular and extracurricular activities and manifested in their academic performance, are considered.
- attention to individual differences and those of the socioeconomic context in which they develop, based on the elements used to characterize the development process of the IQs and their expression in the educational process in which they participate.
- the relationship between the cognitive and affective aspects, based on the students' experiences from the academic point of view, and the interpersonal relationships that develop during the participation in the training actions, between the participants and the teaching staff.

The researcher, considering that this approach benefits the formative management of the student as the main entity of the teaching-learning process, is oriented towards the academic performance of the students for whom the methodological strategy for the development of CI is designed and shown.

Technological: The author considers that, from the perspective of this research, even though this foundation is implicit as a dynamic element of the ALFIN process by promoting the use of computer and information resources for the search, selection, organization, analysis and communication of scientific information, it constitutes an indispensable element for the profession.

Therefore, it is necessary to use them in a conscious way, which favors the development of knowledge, skills and behaviors in the use and access to ICT, while enabling an efficient management of scientific information and knowledge, based on the number of formats, media and digital resources that exist. Therefore, the strengthening of the use of ICTs within the methodological strategy should be emphasized.

In the ALFIN training process, in the methodological strategy designed, ICTs play a fundamental role, including the gamification that is deployed in workshops, the use of the virtual health classroom, trainings and other activities that are presented as part of the process, in which students put into practice their knowledge with the use of playful tools to achieve a specific objective.

It is also evidenced in the methodological actions and procedures implemented in the methodological strategy and the preparation of teaching-methodological activities, course, workshop and training on ALFIN given to students as part of their preparation in their continuing education, which results in their comprehensive training as professionals. These stated theoretical postulates are conditioned and supported by educational research, its development and the link between the philosophical, sociological, pedagogical, psychological, didactic, technological and legal aspects of the methodological strategy.

Information competencies to be developed with the use of ICTs:

The author assumes the competencies, subcompetencies and indicators stated by Fernández [20] based on the learning outcomes to be achieved with the development of these competencies.

2.3.2. External plane
Stage 1. Sensitization and diagnosis

It constitutes the initial stage of the methodological strategy at the external level. It consists of two phases, awareness and diagnosis. During these phases, the necessary information is obtained to be able to plan and execute the strategy, to subsequently carry out its control, validation, analysis of the results and feedback, in order to improve all the necessary aspects that contribute to making the proposal more robust.

Objectives:

1. To sensitize the academic authorities and students of the Faculty of Health Technology on the need to develop informational skills in students with the use of ICT, in order to provide elements that, from the academy, can contribute to graduate a competent professional in the management of information and knowledge.
2. To determine the state of development of informational competences in the students of the Faculty of Health Technology of the University of Medical Sciences of Havana.
3. Characterize the sample of students involved in the study to obtain an optimal design of the methodological strategy.
4. To determine the learning needs and interests of students in Health Technology careers in relation to ALFIN in academic preparation for efficient information and knowledge management in the teaching-learning process.

Phase 1: Sensitization

Objective:

To sensitize the academic authorities and students of the Faculty of Health Technology on the need to develop informational skills in students with the use of ICT, in order to provide elements that, from the academy, can contribute to graduate a competent professional in the management of information and knowledge.

Methodological actions:

- Hold a meeting with the academic authorities of the Faculty of Health Technology to sensitize them on the need to develop information competencies in students through the use of ICTs.
- Hold a meeting with the students of the Faculty of Health Technology to sensitize them on the need to develop informational competencies with the use

of ICTs to contribute to their professional training, demonstrating their need from curricular and extracurricular activities.

- Develop a motivational workshop with the students where they, based on their experiences, transmit the way they consider most conducive to the development of the methodological strategy, so that the design of the same is adjusted to the expectations of the users.
- Characterize the teaching and technological environment for the implementation of the methodological strategy.

<u>Phase 2: Diagnosis</u>

Objectives:

1. To determine the state of development of informational competences in the students of the Faculty of Health Technology of the University of Medical Sciences of Havana.
2. Characterize the sample of students involved in the study to obtain an optimal design of the methodological strategy.
3. To determine the learning needs and interests of students in Health Technology careers in relation to ALFIN in academic preparation for efficient information and knowledge management in the teaching-learning process.

Methodological actions:

- To apply the instrument for the self-assessment of informational competences using the ALFIN-HUMASS questionnaire adapted by Fernández [20].
- Apply the initial questionnaire to characterize the audience and adjust the activities foreseen in the methodological strategy in order to obtain greater effectiveness and acceptance.
- Hold a meeting with the students of the Faculty of Health Technology to inform them of the objectives, structure and actions planned for the methodological strategy for the development of informational competencies with the use of ICTs.
- Exchange with students about the services provided by the library, the faculty's website, the Cuban Journal of Health Technology and the Havana Journal of

Medical Sciences, belonging to the Faculty of Health Technology and the University of Medical Sciences of Havana, respectively, so that they can be updated about the bibliography and information resources found there, which are very useful for teaching.

- Process the results obtained in the instruments applied to determine the learning needs of the students involved in the research.

- To characterize the initial state of the development of informational competencies in the investigated students based on the initial diagnosis.

- Evaluate with the students the results obtained and their expectations related to the methodological strategy.

- Determine the contents on information competencies needed, based on the professional interests detected in the students in order to include them in the course materials.

- Review the legal documents (PCC Guidelines, RM of the MES, RM 47/2022, the model of the professional, Regulations on the informatization of the country, the programs of disciplines and subjects) to exchange with students on the social requirements regarding information competencies in digital environments.

- To update students in relation to the social requirements concerning information competencies according to legal documentation.

Stage 2. Planning

It constitutes the second stage of the methodological strategy at the external level. It consists of three phases: documentary analysis, organization of contents and virtualization of educational resources. Based on the information gathered in the bibliographic research and the surveys and interviews conducted, a specific methodological strategy will be designed and developed for the development of informational competences in FATESA students at the University of Medical Sciences of Havana.

<u>Objectives:</u>

1. To analyze the legal basis that supports the process of developing information competencies in students with the use of ICT, in order to provide the elements

that, from the academy, can contribute to graduate a competent professional in the management of information and knowledge.

2. To determine the contents and their organization in order to promote the development of informational competences in the students of the Faculty of Health Technology of the University of Medical Sciences of Havana through the subject, taking into consideration the results of the diagnosis carried out.

3. Updating of the contents in order to provide the student with knowledge based on the daily reality and related to the professional environment in which he/she works in education at work, so that he/she achieves an adequate relationship between the necessary knowledge for the development of his/her skills, professional attitudes and necessary values in relation to the management of information and knowledge.

4. Virtualization of contents in the Virtual Health Classroom, in order to increase the use of ICTs in the teaching-learning process.

5. Development of digital content for the teaching-learning process of the subject.

Phase 1: Documentary analysis

Objectives:

1. To analyze the legal basis that supports the process of developing information competencies in students with the use of ICT, in order to provide the elements that, from the academy, can contribute to graduate a competent professional in the management of information and knowledge.

Methodological actions:

- Analyze RM 47/2022 and the instructions in force for the undergraduate program, the objectives, methods, means, organizational forms and evaluation that will be developed during the process of development of informational competencies through the subject Informational competencies and collaborative work environments in network.

- Review of the programs of the Integrating Core Discipline, of the subject education at work, skills cards for education at work, teaching-methodological plan, educational project and program of the subject information competencies and collaborative work environments in network.

<u>Phase 2: Organization of contents</u>

Objectives:

1. To determine the contents and their organization in order to promote the development of informational competences in the students of the Faculty of Health Technology of the University of Medical Sciences of Havana through the subject, taking into consideration the results of the diagnosis carried out.

2. To update the contents in order to provide the student with knowledge based on the daily reality and related to the professional environment in which he/she works, so that he/she achieves an adequate relationship between the necessary knowledge for the development of his/her skills, professional attitudes and necessary values in relation to the management of information and knowledge.

Methodological actions:

- Review of the programs of the Integrating Major Discipline, work education plan, work education skills cards, teaching-methodological plan, educational project and subject program.
- Based on the existing possibilities, modify the contents of the program to adjust them to the needs of the students that were identified in the diagnosis, as well as taking into account the latest educational technologies. [86-88].
- Content organization according to the topics foreseen in the course syllabus and the informational competences to be developed.
- Determine the different organizational forms and the didactic components to be used in each of them, the informational resources and bibliography.
- Determine the infotechnological tools and resources to be used in the methodological strategy.

- Select the teaching-learning means, the human and informational resources that will support the methodological actions, such as scientific databases, the Internet, computers, bibliography, librarians, among others.
- Check the operation of the computers in the laboratory, connections, Internet access, availability of databases and the established schedule.

Phase 3: Virtualization of educational resources

Objectives:

1. Virtualize the contents of the Virtual Health Classroom in order to increase the use of ICTs in the teaching-learning process.
2. Develop digital content for the teaching-learning process of the subject.

Methodological actions:

- Determine the infotechnological tools and resources to be used in the methodological strategy.
- Updating of the contents and incorporation of new activities and resources in the Virtual Health Classroom course.
- Content organization according to the topics foreseen in the course syllabus and the informational competencies to be developed in the Virtual Health Classroom.
- Determine the different organizational forms and the didactic components to be used in each of them, the informational resources and bibliography in digital format within the Virtual Health Classroom.
- Development of teaching materials, control questions and design of evaluation activities from the Virtual Health Classroom.

Stage 3. Execution and control

It constitutes the third stage of the proposed methodological strategy. In this stage, the implementation and evaluation of the contents included in the strategy are developed. It is composed of two phases: execution and control. In the first phase, the designed methodological strategy will be implemented in a group of students of the faculty, who will receive training and support in the use of the technological tools and resources proposed from the subject information competences and collaborative network environments. Subsequently, in the second phase, the impact of the strategy on the development of students' information competencies will be evaluated through various indicators, such as the improvement of the use of ICT in the teaching-learning process for the formation of information competencies, the creation of digital resources, participation in virtual communities, among others.

Objectives:

1. To teach the subject Information competencies and collaborative network environments to fourth year students of the regular daytime course of the Health Information Systems career as a selected sample.
2. Execute all methodological actions foreseen in the strategy.
3. To enable and use the information exchange channels between the teacher and the students, as a way of using ICT to facilitate the process of developing information competencies through mobile technology.
4. Evaluate the development of information competencies through evaluation and monitoring activities based on academic performance and visits to education areas at work.
5. Develop skills in the practical area, which will be evaluated through the skills assessment card for on-the-job education.

Phase 1: Execution

Objectives:

1. To teach the subject Information competencies and collaborative network environments to fourth year students of the regular daytime course of the Health Information Systems career as a selected sample.
2. Execute all methodological actions foreseen in the strategy.
3. To enable and use the information exchange channels between the teacher and the students, as a way of using ICT to facilitate the process of developing information competencies through mobile technology.

Methodological actions:

- Determine the infotechnological tools and resources to be used in the methodological strategy.
- Updating of the contents and incorporation of new activities and resources in the Virtual Health Classroom course.
- Content organization according to the topics foreseen in the course syllabus and the informational competencies to be developed in the Virtual Health Classroom.
- Determine the different organizational forms and the didactic components to be used in each of them, the informational resources and bibliography in digital format within the Virtual Health Classroom.
- Apply tools and information resources such as bibliographic managers (Zotero, Endnote, Mendeley, among others) for the organization, retrieval and use of bibliography as technology to support the PEA and the use of Google Scholar to create profiles, libraries, alerts for monitoring a specific topic, perform searches, retrieve them, reference and cite recognized authors.
- Execute the organizational forms that were planned, the practical and theoretical activities foreseen for the development of information competencies.

<u>Phase 2: Control</u>

Objectives:

1. Evaluate the development of information competencies through evaluation and monitoring activities based on academic performance and visits to education areas in the workplace.
2. Develop skills in the practical area, which will be evaluated through the skills assessment card for on-the-job education.

Methodological actions:

- Development of monitoring and evaluation activities in the Virtual Health Classroom.
- Information to students of the schedule of rotations in on-the-job education and indication of the skills to be developed in them.
- Execution of activities to control education in the workplace.

- Evaluation of performance in the areas where students carry out on-the-job education activities, with emphasis on the use of information technology tools and ICTs to solve problems in the work environment.
- Evaluation of the contents taught in the course according to the planning established in the syllabus of the subject, promoting the use of ICT for the solution of the proposed exercises.
- Concretize the evaluation, which should be carried out systematically, so that students appropriate the knowledge, skills and behaviors for the development of an information culture, using the various forms of evaluation.
- Carry out a final theoretical and practical exercise in which students demonstrate the knowledge and competencies developed during the course.

Stage 4. Evaluation and feedback

This is the last stage of the proposed methodological strategy. It will include the analysis of the results obtained from the implementation and evaluation of the methodological strategy, in order to identify strengths, weaknesses and possible improvements for future implementations. Likewise, the results obtained will be disseminated and socialized through scientific articles, presentations in congresses and seminars, and publications in specialized journals, with the objective of contributing to the knowledge and development of information competencies in the university environment from the undergraduate level.

The evaluation fulfills a diagnostic, formative and control function, it will be used in its different modalities: evaluation, co-evaluation and self-evaluation, to issue the value criteria in the fulfillment of the objectives proposed in the subject and the proposed methodological activities. It is necessary to specify that the evaluation will be during the whole process, before, during and after, thus guaranteeing continuous feedback and the fulfillment of the objective.

This stage consists of two phases: evaluation and feedback.

<u>Objectives:</u>

1. Systematically evaluate each of the stages and phases of the process in terms of the knowledge, skills, behaviors and values that students have acquired during their continuous education within the development of the subject.
2. Diagnose the improvement and development of the expected information competencies.
3. Evaluate the level of satisfaction with the development of the methodological strategy based on the contents, use of ICT, organization of contents and activities, among other aspects.
4. Validate the strategy based on the criteria of experts.
5. Adapt the contents, stages, phases and actions based on the results achieved in order to obtain qualitatively superior results in future editions.

<u>Phase 1: Evaluation</u>

Objectives:

1. Systematically evaluate each of the stages and phases of the process in terms of the knowledge, skills, behaviors and values that students have acquired during their continuous education within the development of the subject.
2. Diagnose the improvement and development of the expected information competencies.
3. Evaluate the level of satisfaction with the development of the methodological strategy based on the contents, use of ICT, organization of contents and activities, among other aspects.

Methodological actions:

- Analysis of the results obtained by the students during the development of the course.
- Analysis of the results obtained by students during on-the-job education.
- Post-course application of the ALFIN-HUMASS information literacy self-assessment questionnaire adapted by Fernández. [20].
- Application of the satisfaction survey.

<u>Phase 2: Feedback</u>

Objectives:

1. Validate the strategy based on the criteria of experts.
2. Adapt the contents, stages, phases and actions based on the results achieved in order to obtain qualitatively superior results in future editions.

Methodological actions:

- Determination of the social relevance of the proposed methodological strategy.
- Validation of the methodological strategy by experts.
- Validation of the instruments to be applied by experts.
- Updating of the strategy based on the results achieved during its execution and validation.

2.3.3. Contextual level

This plane is characterized by the development of informational competences with the use of ICT. It is demonstrated after the analysis of the results achieved during the systematic and final evaluation of the development of informational competences by the students both in the scenario of the university classroom, the virtual classroom and the performance area of education at work.

Conclusions of the chapter

The theoretical references that support the implementation of the proposed methodological strategy were described. The operational definition of the methodological strategy with the use of information and communication technologies for the development of informational competences in the students of the Faculty of Health Technology of the University of Medical Sciences of Havana was carried out. The proposed methodological strategy was modeled. The proposed strategy was also described.

CHAPTER 3: IMPLEMENTATION AND EVALUATION OF RESULTS

Chapter III. Implementation and evaluation of results

Introduction to the chapter

This chapter deals with the implementation process of the methodological strategy. To this end, the results obtained after applying the diagnosis and the initial questionnaire for the characterization of the audience, the characterization of the implementation environment, as well as the results achieved by the students during the development of the strategy are discussed. The proposed methodological strategy is described and the results of the validations by experts of the instruments applied and of the strategy itself are also presented, as well as the results of the satisfaction survey of the students who took the course with the implemented strategy.

3.1 Initial diagnosis of informational competencies with the use of information and communication technologies in undergraduate students of the Faculty of Health Technology of the University of Medical Sciences of Havana.

3.1.1. Design of the initial diagnosis

The initial diagnosis was carried out through the ALFIN-HUMASS competency self-assessment questionnaire adapted by Fernández [20]. This questionnaire is designed to know the opinion about knowledge and skills in the processing and use of information. In it, the student will indicate his/her evaluation of the following skills by circling the one that best expresses his/her answer, on a scale from 1 (lowest) to 9 (excellent). The student will also evaluate each skill in relation to three variables (motivational commitment, self-efficacy, and source of learning).

3.1.2. Assessment of the results of the initial diagnosis

For the analysis of the indicators "commitment to motivation" and "self-efficacy", the median was used as a summary measure. In the case of "source of learning", the mode was used. In this way we avoided bias due to the presence of outliers or incongruent values within the observation, based on the answers provided by the respondents.

The following scale was used to interpret the data:

1 Low; 2-3 Medium Low; 4-6 Medium; 7-8 Medium High and 9 High

The overall results of the initial diagnosis are shown in Table 1, which shows the indicators grouped according to the measures of central tendency declared, grouped by the four categories of knowledge and skills presented in the instrument applied.

Table 1. Results of the initial diagnosis

Regarding...	Motivation commitment	Self-efficiency	Source of learning
Knowledge-Skills	**Low High** **1 2 3 4 5 6 7 8 9**	**Low High** **1 2 3 4 5 6 7 8 9**	**Cl - Classes - 1 Co - Courses - 2 B - Library - 3 A - Self-preparation - 4 O - Others - 5**
Information Search	6,0	6,0	1,0
Evaluation of information	8,0	8,0	1,0
Information processing	6,0	7,0	1,0
Communication and dissemination of information	5,0	6,0	1,0

Regarding the criterion "commitment to motivation", there is a tendency to a medium evaluation, three of the four indicators are found with values between 4 and 6, with the evaluation of information as the knowledge/skill that most motivates the students standing out in the medium-high category.

In the case of self-efficacy, there is a tendency to a better evaluation by the students, two of the criteria obtain a medium rating, while the remaining two obtain a medium-high rating. In this aspect, the knowledge/skills where the students appreciate a higher self-efficacy are evaluation and information processing.

Regarding the source of learning, there is consensus that the knowledge/skills studied are acquired in the classroom.

3.2. Characterization of students according to the initial competency questionnaire

The sample studied was composed of 29 students, of whom 13 were male and 16 were female, with the female sex predominating with a ratio of 1.23 female to male within the sample.

The average age is 22 years, all of them being students coming from pre-university. In this aspect it is worth mentioning that only a minority, 4 (15%) passed the entrance exams and applied for the career they are studying from the first call, so that the motivation towards the professional profile is an element to work hard during each subject and academic year.

The totality of the sample responded that they have internet connection, 10.3% (3) do it less than one hour a day, 13.8% (4) do it between one and five hours and 75.9% (22) do it more than 5 hours.

Within the use of the Internet, among the options offered, the use of the Internet for reading for studying and interaction with social networks stood out, with 24 students in both options, which represented 82.8% in each of them with respect to the total surveyed. Next in descending order were the options of watching videos for distraction and instructional videos, with 22 students, which represented 75.9% in each aspect surveyed. The category with the lowest incidence was playing games, with 4 students, for 13.8%.

With regard to knowledge of information literacy as a method of training and development of information competencies, only five students responded positively, which represented 17.2%.

Regarding knowledge of virtual teaching and learning environments, 86.2% responded affirmatively, and these were the same as those who said they were familiar with the Virtual Health Classroom.

Regarding the skills surveyed, information search and processing were the only ones in which all the students stated that they had skills. Of the rest of the items surveyed, those related to recognition and respect for the work and ideas expressed by other authors with 82.8% and learning through digital environments with 86.2% of affirmative responses with respect to the total surveyed stood out for having a high percentage of affirmative responses.

These results corroborated the self-assessment of competencies carried out by the students when answering the diagnostic questionnaire using the ALFIN-HUMASS instrument.

3.3. Characterization of the implementation environment

The Faculty of Health Technology of the University of Medical Sciences of Havana is located at Carvajal Street # 155 / A and Agua Dulce, Cerro municipality. It is a provincial faculty and receives students from some municipalities of the provinces of Artemisa and Mayabeque. It is the National Methodological Rector Center for Health Technology careers. For the implementation of the methodological strategy it has:

- Medical Library equipped with 10 computers with Internet connectivity. The printed document collection is poor and mostly outdated. Since the pandemic, the library has not provided the usual services, mainly due to the lack of specialized human resources and the damage to the teaching infrastructure after the passage of Hurricane Ian, which caused the library to be used as a teaching scenario for the Health Information Systems career to replace the classrooms affected by the meteorological event.
- Computer laboratories, two for all careers, except Health Information Systems, which, as it is part of the discipline, has its own two laboratories, all equipped and with Internet connectivity.

Two scenarios were selected for on-the-job education:

- Library of the Calixto García School of Medical Sciences, with little equipment, but with connectivity in which it has a printed documentary collection with a good degree of updating, mainly in theses of different purposes and with qualified, specialized and teaching category human resources.
- Library of the Salvador Allende School of Medical Sciences, adjacent to FATESA, with qualified personnel, little equipment, but with connectivity and space and conditions for the development of information competencies.

3.4. Implementation of the methodological strategy for the development of informational competencies with the use of information and communication technologies in undergraduate students of the Faculty of Health Technology of the University of Medical Sciences of Havana.

3.4.1. Implementation Design

The implementation of the methodological strategy was carried out in the Health Information Systems course, using, as already stated, a sample of 27 students who took the course "Information competencies and collaborative work environments in networks".

The initial sample was divided into two groups, faithfully adjusted to the distribution designated by the teaching secretary. The first group, SIS 41, with a total of 12 students and SIS 42 with 17 students. The initial diagnosis and the initial questionnaire were carried out with this sample.

During the course of the research, there were two withdrawals from the research sample, both from the second group (SIS 42), both because they dropped out of the course, one of them because he left the country and the other because of family problems, who did not request a leave of absence. The final sample, with which the validation of the research and final diagnosis was carried out, consisted of 27 students, organized in the two academic groups of the career, SIS 41 with 12 students and SIS 42 with 15.

The final gender distribution was 12 males and 15 females, with a predominance of females with a ratio of 1.25 females to males in the sample.

The implementation period was the 2022 academic year, in the second semester.

3.4.2. Execution of implementation

As mentioned above, the methodological strategy was implemented in the subject of information competencies and collaborative work environments in the network, which has 8 teaching topics in the update that addresses the training and development of information competencies. The program includes 120 hours of face-to-face classes and is complemented by 114 hours of on-the-job education and 46 hours of independent work, together with 4 hours dedicated to the final theoretical-practical exam, for a total of 234 hours and an extension of 17 teaching weeks.

The main contents addressed are related to information literacy, development of critical thinking, information competences, information metric studies, Web 2.0 paradigm, Content Management Systems (CMS) to share information and knowledge (Wiki, Blogs and others), Virtual Environments for corporate work in NETWORK (Plone, Drupal and others as technological platform. Installation and configuration of services) and finally Virtual Environments for Teaching and Learning. Moodle as a technological platform. Installation and configuration.

The course is available in the Virtual Health Classroom, in the work area of the Faculty of Health Technology FATESA, corresponding to the Health Information Systems Career according to the academic year and semester in which it is taught.

In the virtual course topics were enabled according to those planned in the program of the subject, within each one can be found activities such as Forums, Quizzes, Tasks, folders with the recommended bibliography, teaching materials and presentations, Wiki, Workshop, among other resources and activities that the Moodle platform allows.

Collaterally, a second course was enabled where students acquire the role of teacher, in which they put into practice all the knowledge acquired during the course within the topic dedicated to each one of them. This space is mainly dedicated to the development of the skills of Topic 8, although it is oriented to plan the activities taking into account the knowledge and skills acquired throughout the course.

The final exam of the course consists of a theoretical-practical exam, in which students answer an integrative questionnaire from the AVS and in the practical area develop the exercises indicated in a randomly chosen ballot.

For the proper implementation of all the activities planned in the methodological strategy, a WhatsApp group was set up for the exchange of information, comments and initiatives between teachers and students, as well as to develop skills using mobile technology, as this is the most common means of access through which students connect to the AVS.

ICTs were used for the development of the subject itself, as a means of communication and as a work tool, by using infotechnological tools for the development of informational competencies in students.

3.5. Validation of the methodological strategy for the development of informational competencies with the use of information and communication technologies in undergraduate students of the Faculty of Health Technology of the University of Medical Sciences of Havana.

3.5.1. Validation strategy

Four validation moments were established, each characterized by the content and the subjects involved in the process. The validation strategy was designed through consultation with specialists (using expert judgment) for the instruments applied (initial questionnaire and satisfaction survey) as well as the proposed methodological strategy; user satisfaction; student academic performance results; and finally the application of the ALFIN-HUMASS competency self-assessment questionnaire (beginning and end of the study).

3.5.2. Validation by consultation with specialists using expert judgement

Specialists were consulted on three occasions. On each occasion, the instrument designed by Escobar and Cuervo [89] was used to explore [89] for content validation by expert judgment.

Five specialists were interviewed three times, the first time to evaluate the initial competency questionnaire, the second time to validate the proposed methodological strategy and the third time to validate the satisfaction survey , all of whom have a high level of knowledge about IQ and academic performance. The selection requirements for the specialists were:

- to be a university professor
- consent of each one to participate
- be linked to the scientific activity being investigated

The specialists agreed to participate voluntarily and anonymously in the evaluation of the methodological strategy and the instruments requested, a willingness that they expressed in the Informed Consent form.

After their consent to participate as specialists, they were sent by e-mail or by personal delivery the instruments designed for the validation of the contents of the initial competency questionnaire, the methodological strategy and the satisfaction survey.

3.5.2.1. Validation by consultation with specialists using expert judgment of the initial questionnaire

In the initial questionnaire for characterizing the sample and determining the information competencies they possess, 12 indicators related to the ICs to be developed were measured, with sufficiency, coherence, relevance and clarity as evaluation indicators. In each aspect, the expert should record a score between 1 and 4 points for each attribute, where 1 means little or none and 4 means a lot. In case the score is lower than 3, the expert should justify in the comments section the reasons he/she considers.

The aspects evaluated were grouped according to the dimensions determined for the analysis of the variable, which were informational knowledge, informational skills, informational attitudes and informational aptitudes.

The evaluation by the experts generally showed positive results, which could be verified not only by the descriptive evaluation of the answers, but also through non-parametric statistical tests.

Nonparametric statistical methods were used to evaluate the concordance of the responses of all the specialists consulted. The following hypotheses were put forward:

H_0 : there is agreement among the experts as to the coherence, relevance, clarity and sufficiency of the aspects evaluated for the initial competency questionnaire.

H_1 : there is no agreement among the experts as to the coherence, relevance, clarity and sufficiency of the aspects evaluated for the initial competency questionnaire.

Since these are independent samples, the Kruskal-Wallis test for independent samples will be performed, taking into account the following assumptions:

1. The data do not follow a normal distribution.

Confidence interval: 95%.

3. Significance level: 0.05.

When evaluating the results after applying the Kolmogorov-Smirnov test, significant statistics are obtained, P-Value (Coherence), P-Value (Relevance), P-Value (Clarity) and P-Value (Sufficiency) in all the questions evaluated reflect values less than 0.05, so the null hypothesis is rejected and it is concluded that the data do not conform to a normal distribution. Taking this into account, parametric tests cannot be used.

Therefore, it was decided to apply the Kruskal-Wallis test for independent samples. When evaluating the values of asymptotic significance, values greater than 0.05 are obtained in all the questions evaluated, therefore, the null hypothesis is not rejected and it is concluded that there is agreement among the experts regarding the coherence, relevance, clarity and sufficiency of the aspects evaluated for the methodological strategy.

3.5.2.2. Validation of the methodological strategy by consulting specialists using expert judgment.

The methodological strategy for its application in this research considered the author to carry out its validation, through the instrument designed for this purpose, in order to comply with the essential metric attributes for its use - reliability and validity - with the purpose of carrying out the validation of content: sufficiency, clarity, coherence and relevance.

The aspects subjected to expert appraisal were as follows:

- Objectives of the methodological strategy
- Structure of the methodological strategy
- Correspondence between the objectives of each phase, stage and general
- Organization of methodological actions
- Fundamentals of the methodological strategy
- Correspondence between the methodological actions and the informational competencies to be developed.

The opinion of the specialists who evaluated the methodological strategy coincides in the majority, with respect to the attributes measured with a high score, in the feasibility of the methodological activities planned to develop IQ in the students.

However, some felt that modifications should be made in terms of incorporating educational trends as technology develops, which would help improve students' development of IQs .

Nonparametric statistical methods were used to evaluate the concordance of the responses of all the specialists consulted. The following hypotheses were put forward:

H_0 : there is agreement among the experts as to the coherence, relevance, clarity and sufficiency of the aspects evaluated for the methodological strategy.

H_1 : there is no agreement among the experts regarding the coherence, relevance, clarity and sufficiency of the aspects evaluated for the methodological strategy.

Since we are dealing with independent samples, the Kruskal-Wallis test for independent samples will be performed, taking into account the following assumptions:

1. The data do not follow a normal distribution.

Confidence interval: 95%.

3. Significance level: 0.05.

When evaluating the results after applying the Kolmogorov-Smirnov test, significant statistics are obtained, P-Value (Coherence), P-Value (Relevance), P-Value (Clarity) and P-Value (Sufficiency) in all the questions evaluated reflect values less than 0.05, so the null hypothesis is rejected and it is concluded that the data do not conform to a normal distribution. Taking this into account, parametric tests cannot be used.

Therefore, it was decided to apply the Kruskal-Wallis test for independent samples. When evaluating the values of asymptotic significance, values greater than 0.05 are obtained in all the questions evaluated, therefore, the null hypothesis is not rejected and it is concluded that there is agreement among the experts regarding the coherence, relevance, clarity and sufficiency of the aspects evaluated for the methodological strategy.

3.5.2.3. Validation by consultation with specialists using expert judgment of the satisfaction survey

The satisfaction survey was evaluated by the specialists, all of whom were of the opinion that it complies with the attributes measured: coherence, relevance and clarity, aspects measured in the instrument applied for its evaluation.

Nonparametric statistical methods were used to evaluate the concordance of the responses of all the specialists consulted. The following hypotheses were put forward:

H_0 : there is agreement among the experts on the consistency, relevance and clarity of the satisfaction survey questions.

H_1 : there is no agreement among the experts on the consistency, relevance and clarity of the satisfaction survey questions.

Since these are independent samples, the Kruskal-Wallis test will be performed, taking into account the following assumptions:

1. The data do not follow a normal distribution.

Confidence interval: 95%.

3. Significance level: 0.05.

To start the test we checked that the data do not comply with a normal distribution. When evaluating the results after applying the Kolmogorov-Smirnov test we obtain significant statistics, P-Value (Coherence), P-Value (Relevance) and P-Value (Clarity) in all the evaluated questions less than 0.05 so we reject the null hypothesis and conclude that the data do not conform to a normal distribution. Taking this into account, parametric tests cannot be used.

Therefore, it was decided to apply the Kruskal-Wallis test for independent samples. When evaluating the values of asymptotic significance, values greater than 0.05 were obtained for all the questions evaluated; therefore, the null hypothesis is not rejected and it is concluded that there is agreement among the experts regarding the coherence, relevance and clarity of the questions in the satisfaction survey.

3.5.3. Validation by level of user satisfaction .

For validation by level of user satisfaction, the Likert scale was applied in a 7-question survey with a 3- and 5-point scale. The satisfaction survey was applied to the 27 students who constituted the final sample of the study, since two students dropped out of the research.

The Likert scale, named after its developer, Rensis Likert, invented in the 1930s, is a popularly used rating scale that requires respondents to indicate the degree of agreement or disagreement with each of a series of statements about stimulus objects. Odd and even measurement scales are established, and the 5-point Likert scale and the 7-point Likert scale with a midpoint are much more commonly used in questionnaires and surveys [90].

An important benefit of Likert-type questions is their flexibility, as they can be used to collect information on sentiment toward a wide range of topics. Some typical survey response scales are as follows. [90]:

Agreement: Assess the extent to which respondents agree or disagree with statements or opinions.

Value: To measure the perceived worth or importance of something.

Relevance: To measure the relevance or suitability of specific elements or content.

Frequency: Determine how often certain events or behaviors occur.

Importance: Evaluate the importance or significance of various factors or criteria.

Quality: Evaluate the level of quality of products, services or experiences.

Probability: Estimating the likelihood of future events or behaviors.

Measure: To measure the extent to which something is true or applicable.

Competence: To assess the perceived competence or skills of individuals or organizations.

Comparison: Compare and rank preferences or opinions.

Performance: Evaluate the performance or effectiveness of systems, processes or individuals.

Satisfaction: Measure how satisfied and dissatisfied someone is with the product and service.

For the instrument designed for the research, those related to satisfaction were used. To evaluate the results, 3-point and 5-point questions were used, in the case of the topics addressed, they were satisfaction, probability, value and measurement.

Satisfaction scale:

Very satisfied - 5; Satisfied - 4; Neither satisfied nor dissatisfied - 3; Not satisfied - 2; Not satisfied - 1.

Probability scale:

Definitely will - 5; Probably will - 4; Don't know - 3; Probably won't - 2; Definitely won't - 1.

Scale of measurement:

Extremely - 5; Very well - 4; Moderately - 3; Slightly - 2; Not at all - 1.

Value scale:

Very positive - 5; Positive - 4; Neither positive nor negative - 3; Negative - 2; Very negative - 1.

The 3-item question was designed using as possible answers: Yes, No and Don't know.

The student satisfaction survey can be implemented from the application of the instrument, the following results were obtained:

The degree of satisfaction expressed with the course in general is valued by the students as satisfied (4), a value obtained as average, median and mode. This value was contributed by 51.9% of the students, followed by the category very satisfied (5) which was referred by 33.3%.

The degree of satisfaction with the contents taught showed results similar to those evaluated in the previous item. Among the negative values, only 1 student (3.7%) reported feeling dissatisfied, while 3 others (11.1%) gave a neutral evaluation, reporting feeling neither satisfied nor dissatisfied.

The degree of satisfaction with the use of ICT in the development process of the subject is positively evaluated, with 16 evaluations of satisfied (59.3%) and 10 of very satisfied (37.0%).

Regarding the probability of applying the knowledge acquired for academic and professional performance, 13 students stated that they would definitely do so, which represented 48.1% of the total of the final sample, while 12 others (44.4%) stated that they would probably do so, which translates into a positive evaluation based on the consideration that the knowledge acquired could be useful in their performance.

When asked about the development of informational competencies through the subject using the applied methodological strategy, 16 students (59.2%) stated that they did extremely well, while 8 (29.6%) marked the category very well. No student reported negativity in this question.

Regarding the influence of ICT in the process of developing information competencies, 15 students (55.5%) stated that they considered the influence to be very positive, while the remaining 12 (45.5%) stated that it was positive.

To evaluate the concordance of the results obtained, nonparametric statistical methods were applied. The following hypotheses were proposed:

H_0 : there is concordance in the level of satisfaction with the methodological strategy used between the two groups.

H_1 : there is no concordance in the level of satisfaction with the methodological strategy used between the two groups.

Since these are independent samples, the Mann-Withney U test will be performed, taking into account the following assumptions:

    1. The data do not follow a normal distribution.

Confidence interval: 95%.

3. Significance level: 0.05.

To start the test we checked that the data do not comply with a normal distribution. When evaluating the results after applying the Kolmogorov-Smirnov test we obtain significant statistics, P-Value (SIS41) and P-Value (SIS42) in all the evaluated questions less than 0.05 so we reject the null hypothesis and conclude that the data do not conform to a normal distribution. Taking this into account, parametric tests cannot be used.

Therefore, it was decided to apply the Mann-Whitney U test for independent samples. When evaluating the values of asymptotic significance (bilateral), values greater than 0.05 are obtained in all the questions evaluated, so the null hypothesis is not rejected and it is concluded that there is concordance in the level of satisfaction with the methodological strategy used between the two groups.

Validation by academic results achieved by the students during the implementation of the methodological strategy.

An important element to corroborate the effectiveness of the methodological strategy is the evaluation of the students' academic performance during the course of the subject. For this reason, the researcher decided to carry out this type of validation.

The final results of the subject Information competencies and collaborative network environments, which were analyzed qualitatively and quantitatively, were taken into account. It should be noted that 100% of the students passed the course, 24 of them in the ordinary theoretical-practical exam and 3 in the first extraordinary exam.

With an evaluation of Excellent (5 points), 5 students from the SIS 41 and SIS 42 groups were evaluated, respectively, for a total of 10 students evaluated with this grade. With an evaluation of Good (4 points), 7 students from SIS 41 and 10 from SIS 42 were evaluated.

Descriptively, it can be concluded that, of the 27 students sampled, 10 achieved an Excellent evaluation, which represented 37% of the total, while the remaining 63% obtained a grade of Good.

To evaluate this result using nonparametric statistics, the following hypotheses were proposed:

H_0 : the average evaluation in each group was 4 points (Good).

H_1 : the average evaluation in each group was different from 4 points (Good).

Since these are independent samples, the Mann-Withney U test will be performed, taking into account the following assumptions:

1. The data do not follow a normal distribution.

Confidence interval: 95%.

3. Significance level: 0.05.

To start the test, we found that the data do not comply with a normal distribution. When evaluating the results after applying the Kolmogorov-Smirnov test, we obtain significant statistics, P-Value (SIS41) and P-Value (SIS42) less than 0.05, so we reject the null hypothesis and conclude that the data do not conform to a normal distribution. Taking this into account, parametric tests cannot be used.

Therefore, it was decided to apply the Mann-Whitney U test for independent samples. When evaluating the values of asymptotic significance (bilateral), values greater than 0.05 are obtained; therefore, the null hypothesis is not rejected and it is concluded that the mean evaluation in each group was 4 points (Good).

3.5.5. Validation according to information competency assessment instrument

In order to validate the instrument for the assessment of information competencies, the ALFIN-HUMASS questionnaire presented by Fernández [20] was used for the second time. [20].

As was done in the case of the initial diagnosis, for the analysis of the indicators "commitment to motivation" and "self-efficacy", the median was used as a summary measure. In the case of "source of learning", the mode was used. In this way we avoided bias due to the presence of outliers or incongruent values within the observation, based on the answers provided by the respondents.

The following scale was used to interpret the data:

1 Low; 2-3 Medium Low; 4-6 Medium; 7-8 Medium High and 9 High

Table 2. Results of the final diagnosis

Regarding...	Motivation commitment	Self-efficiency	Source of learning
Knowledge-Skills	Low High	Low High	Cl - Classes - 1 Co - Courses - 2 B - Library - 3 A - Self-preparation - 4 O - Others - 5
	1 2 3 4 5 6 7 8 9	1 2 3 4 5 6 7 8 9	
Information Search	8,0	8,0	1,0
Evaluation of information	8,0	8,0	1,0
Information processing	9,0	9,0	1,0
Communication and dissemination of information	8,0	8,0	1,0

The overall results of the initial diagnosis are shown in Table 2, which shows the indicators grouped according to the measures of central tendency declared, grouped by the four categories of knowledge and skills presented in the instrument applied.

According to the criterion "commitment to motivation", there is a tendency towards a medium-high valuation, three of the four indicators are found with values of 8, with information processing standing out in the high category as the knowledge/skill that most motivates the students.

In the case of self-efficacy, there is a tendency to a similar evaluation with respect to the previously evaluated element, three of the criteria obtain a medium-high rating, while the remaining one obtained a high rating. In this aspect, the knowledge/skill where the students appreciate a higher self-efficacy is information processing.

Regarding the source of learning, there is consensus that the knowledge/skills studied are acquired in the classroom.

Taking into account the initial diagnosis, the variation between the final and initial evaluations is then analyzed to determine how many points the evaluated elements increased or decreased in the evaluation. The results are shown in Table 3.

Variation between final and initial diagnosis.

Regarding...	Motivation commitment	Self-efficiency	Source of learning
Knowledge-Skills	Low High	Low High	Cl - Classes - 1
	1 2 3 4 5 6 7 8 9	1 2 3 4 5 6 7 8 9	Co - Courses - 2 B - Library - 3 A - Self-preparation - 4 O - Others - 5
Information Search	2,0	2,0	0,0
Evaluation of information	1,0	0,0	0,0
Information processing	3,0	2,0	0,0
Communication and dissemination of information	3,0	2,0	0,0

It is worth noting that in the case of the commitment to motivation is the category with the greatest progress, while the source of learning did not present variation between both evaluation moments. The knowledge/skills with the greatest growth in the evaluations were information processing and communication and dissemination of information.

Conclusions of the chapter

The process of implementation of the methodological strategy was addressed, the results of the initial questionnaire for the characterization of the audience, the characterization of the implementation environment, as well as the results achieved by the students during the development of the strategy were analyzed. Based on the validations by experts of the instruments applied and of the strategy itself, as well as the results of the satisfaction survey of the students who took the course with the implemented strategy and the diagnostics applied before and after the implementation, it is asserted that the methodological strategy meets the proposed objective, so it is also affirmed that it is valid for its future generalization.

GENERAL CONCLUSIONS

Conclusions general

- Information competencies are currently under analysis and need to be approached in a different way in higher and general education.

- The analysis of the scientific literature made it possible to systematize the theoretical and methodological references on the process of developing informational competencies in university students as the object of study in the research and the theoretical cores that integrate it, process, development and informational competencies. It also provided the theoretical references for the field of action determined by the use of ICTs in the process of developing informational competencies. It constituted the basis for the operational definition of the object of study for the research.

- When characterizing the dependent variable, it is shown that there are deficiencies in the development of actions during the teaching-learning process from the curriculum in the development of informational competencies of human resources trained in Health Technology careers at the University of Medical Sciences of Havana, together with the disuse of activities to develop informational competencies through the use of ICTs, reasons that support the need to implement the methodological strategy for the development of informational competencies with the use of ICTs.

- The implemented methodological strategy has three levels in its structure: the internal level (integrated by the objectives, theoretical foundations and informational competences to be developed with the use of ICT) from which emanates the external level that allows the development of the competences integrated by four stages, which in turn are integrated by phases that allow the articulation of methodological actions, manifesting among these relationships of determination, coordination, subordination, hierarchization and complementation. In this sense, various organizational forms and the teaching-methodological work are harmoniously integrated, making it possible for students to achieve an efficient management of information and knowledge. Finally, the contextual level where the development of informational competences is evidenced with the use of ICTs demonstrated by the students who participate in the implementation of the methodological strategy.

- Favorable results are observed in the validation by expert judgment of both the proposed strategy and the instruments used in the research. The diagnostic questionnaires at the beginning and end of the implementation of the methodological strategy show positive results when evaluating the variation between one and the other. The students' academic results are also positive, all of which supports the relevance and effectiveness of the proposal.

RECOMMENDATIONS

Recommendations

- To deepen the research topic through the continuity of professional development in doctoral studies.
- To increase and/or adapt the methodological actions based on the suggestions of the experts and the students' own evaluations, which makes possible the dynamization of the contents taught in the subject Informational competences and collaborative work environments in network.
- Update the methodological strategy every year, taking into account scientific and technological developments (information technology tools, reliable information sources and information resources).
- Extend the methodological strategy adjusted to a teaching program for all the careers of the Faculty of Health Technology.
- To teach the program designed for this purpose in the first year of the degree programs in order to prepare students for optimal academic performance based on the development of information competencies.

BIBLIOGRAPHIC REFERENCES

Bibliographic references

[1] MESA VÁZQUEZ Jorge, María Elena PARDO GÓMEZ and Gardenia Edith CEDEÑO MARCILLO. Informatics and informational competences in scientific information management in postgraduate education. Estudios pedagógicos (Valdivia) [online]. 2022, vol. 48, 103-114.[accessed: 10 March 2023].Available at: http://www.scielo.cl/scielo.php?script=sci_arttext&pid=S0718-07052022000200103&nrm=iso

[2] OLAZABAL GUERRA, Daniel José, Aylin ESTRADA VELAZCO and Yanio HERNÁNDEZ HEREDIA. Information and Communication Technologies in the formation of Informational Competences. Cuban Journal of Health Technology [online]. 2023, 14(4), 1-14 [accessed: 15 November 2023]. ISSN 2218-6719. Available at: https://revtecnologia.sld.cu/index.php/tec/article/view/4058

[3] CHIM MANZANERO, Wendy Gabriela and Alfredo ZAPATA GONZÁLEZ. Digital competencies of secondary level teachers in Ibero-America. A systematic review from 2011 to 2021. Electronic Journal in Education and Pedagogy [online]. 2022, 6(10) [accessed: 21 February 2023]. Available at: doi:10.15658/rev.electron.educ.pedagog22.04061006.

[4] GUTIÉRREZ MARTÍN, Alfonso. Multiple literacy and training in ICT and Media. University Library [online]. 2022, 25(1) [accessed:21 February 2023]. ISSN 2594-0074. Disponible en: doi:http://dx.doi.org/10.22201/dgbsdi.0187750xp.2022.1.1446

[5] SALAZAR FARFÁN, María del Rosario and Galia Susana LESCANO LÓPEZ. Digital competencies in Latin American university teachers: A systematic review. Alpha Centauri [online]. 2022, 3(2), 02-13 [accessed:21 February 2023]. Available at: doi:10.47422/ac.v3i2.69.

[6] GONZÁLEZ CALATAYUD, Victor, Marimar ROMÁN GARCÍA and María Paz PRENDES ESPINOSA. Digital skills training for university students based on the DigComp model. Edutec. Electronic Journal of Educational Technology [online]. 2018, 0(65) [accessed:21 February 2023]. Available at: doi:10.21556/edutec.2018.65.1119.

[7] ALIAGA MARAÑON, Verónica. Information literacy module to consolidate information competencies in students of business administration at a private high school in Lima. [online]. Graduate thesis. Universidad San Ignacio de Loyola, 2022 [accessed: 21 February 2023]. Available at: https://repositorio.usil.edu.pe/items/d6577f06-4f52-4bf1-a318-72f6b73dd670/full

[8] AYUSO, Luis, Félix REQUENA, Olga JIMÉNEZRODRIGUEZ and Nadia KHAMIS. The Effects of COVID-19 Confinement on the Spanish Family: Adaptation or Change? [online]. 2020 [cited: 21 February 2023]. Aviable:https://utpjournals.press/doi/abs/10.3138/jcfs.51.3-4.004

[9] OECD. Making the Most of Technology for Learning and Training in Latin America [online]. 2020 [cited: 21 February 2023]. Aviable: https://www.oecd-ilibrary.org/content/publication/ce2b1a62-en

[10] LAURENTECÁRDENAS, Carlos Miguel, Raúl Alberto RENGIFO-LOZANO, Nicanor Segismundo ASMATVEGA and Lidia NEYRAHUAMANI. Development of digital competencies in university teachers through virtual environments: experiences of university teachers in Lima. Eleuthera [online]. 2020, 22(2), 71-87 [accessed: 21 February 2023]. Available at: doi:10.17151/eleu.2020.22.2.5.

[11] MARIACA GARRON, Magaly Cristit, María Luisa ZAGALAZ SÁNCHEZ, Tomas J. CAMPOY ARANDA and Carmina GONZÁLEZ GONZÁLEZ DE MESA. Bibliographic review on the use of ict in education. International Journal of Social Science Research [online]. 2022, 18, 23-40 [accessed: 21 February 2023]. Available at: http://scielo.iics.una.py/scielo.php?script=sci_arttext&pid=S2226-40002022000100023&nrm=iso

[12] CALLE GONZÁLEZ, Silvia, Karen TORRES BELDUMA and Fernanda TUSA JUMBO. ICTs, teaching and family digital literacy. Transformación [online]. 2022, 18, 94-113 [accessed: 21 February 2023]. Available at: http://scielo.sld.cu/scielo.php?script=sci_arttext&pid=S2077-29552022000100094&nrm=iso

[13] PLASENCIA URIZARRI, Thais María and Luis E. ALMAGUER MEDEROS. Informational competencies in doctoral students of the health sector in Holguin province, Cuba. Habanera Journal of Medical Sciences [online]. 2022, 21 [accessed: 21 February 2023]. Available at: http://scielo.sld.cu/scielo.php?script=sci_arttext&pid=S1729-519X2022000200014&nrm=iso

[14] MAGUIÑA BALLÓN, AndreArmel. Information literacy in the blendedlearning modality in higher education [online]. 2021.-09-01 [accessed: 21 February 2023]. ISBN 1562-4730. Available at: http://biblios.pitt.edu/ojs/index.php/biblios/article/view/859

[15] ALCÍVAR TREJO, Carlos, VARGAS PÁRRAGA, Juan CALDERÓN CISNEROS, Carlos TRIVIÑO IBARRA, Sara SANTILLÁN INDACOCHEA, Roberto SORIA VERA and Laura CÁRDENAS ZUMA. The use of ICT in the teaching-learning process of teachers in the Universities of Ecuador. Espacios [online]. 2019, 40(2), 27[accessed: 24 February 2023]. ISSN 0798 1015. Available at: https://www.revistaespacios.com/a19v40n02/19400227.html

[16] PUIG MENESES, Yaima. From the informatization of society to digital transformation in Cuba. Presidency and Government of Cuba [online]. 2021 [accessed: 11 March 2023]. Available at: https://www.presidencia.gob.cu/es/noticias/de-la-informatizacion-de-la-sociedad-a-la-transformacion-digital-en-cuba/

[17]   REDACCIÓN MINSAP. How is the informatization process in the health sector progressing? Ministry of Public Health Republic of Cuba [online]. 2019 [accessed: 11 March 2023]. Available at: https://salud.msp.gob.cu/como-marcha-el-proceso-de-informatizacion-en-el-sector-de-la-salud/

[18]   GUTIERREZ VERA, Dayami, Miday COLUMBIÉ PILETA, Tania Rosa GARCIA GONZALEZ, Lisandra DUANY OSORIA, Nadia Marisol SANTIZO PITTO and Eloy MORASEN ROBLES. Informational skills with focus on health information systems. Cuban Journal of Health Technology [online]. 2020, 11(1), 8 [accessed: 10 October 2023]. ISSN 2218-6719. Available at: https://revtecnologia.sld.cu/index.php/tec/article/view/1780

[19]   ZELADA PÉREZ, Malena. Curricular model for the development of informational competencies in teachers of the University of Medical Sciences of Havana [online]. Havana, 2018 [accessed: 11 March 2023]. Doctoral dissertation. University of Medical Sciences of Havana. Available at: http://tesis.sld.cu/index.php/index.php?P=FullRecord&ID=681

[20]   FERNÁNDEZ VALDÉS, María de las Mercedes. El desarrollo de competencias informacionales en ciencias de la salud a partir del paradigma de la transdisciplinariedad. A formative proposal. [online]. Granada, Spain, Havana, Cuba, 2013 [accessed: 11 March 2023]. Doctoral Thesis. University of Granada and University of Havana. Disponible en: http://tesis.sld.cu/index.php?P=FullRecord&ID=211&ReturnText=Search+Results&ReturnTo=index.php%3FP%3DAdvancedSearch%26Q%3DY%26G100%3D1028%26RP%3D5%26SR%3D5%26SF%3D84%26SD%3D1

[21]   ROYAL SPANISH ACADEMY. Diccionario de la Lengua Española [online]. 2022 [accessed: 11 March 2023]. Available at: https://dle.rae.es

[22]   MALDONADO, José Ángel. Process management [online]. 2018 [accessed: 03 October 2023]. Available from: https://d1wqtxts1xzle7.cloudfront.net/55606149/GESTION_DE_PROCESOS_2018-libre.pdf?1516650790=&response-content-disposition=inline%3B+filename%3DPROCESS_MANAGEMENT.pdf&Expires=1696376930&Signature=bPxkTUM7GdClLAbJ5A3Ah5VwXYlEt-QykedCVkG-9cYFIHM9Hj3DLgiIqKsUVvxTqjcAFwfLjnrMjzJ0xXpc1CPI00VnvaH4t1fcOhXWeziNzf3FDibzqFa~jJdV4ig3M--jfQbN92o-qj2yxiUwWNUNs5Bh0fk1AozwsO9RQe1VQEUW~utjpFuzM9s1Pz6mv4n005GXnx3FV5QkIZzvEEg92s6ibELjAuidhx2T24uUMWSCclT0rPsq8~LPE8tMqCdWVVkx~V2g9SdWAamuJwNvRrIqbZso3rQ-LjmVkLFGfMvzs91Z5f9-Gxlm-cj2yqsTbAJwRL5NVbFjb~465Rw__&&Key-Pair-Id=APKAJLOHF5GGSLRBV4ZA

[23]   ISO 9000:2005 Quality management systems [online]. 2005 [accessed: 03 October 2023]. Available at: https://www.iso.org/obp/ui/#iso:std:iso:9000:ed-3:v1:es:term:3.2.5

[24] DUBOIS, Alfonso. A concept of development for the 21st century. Journal of economic and administrative affairs [online]. 2002, 8, 1-11 [accessed: 11 November 2023]. Available at: https://www.institutodeestudiosglobales.org/resources/Un%20concepto%20de%20desarrollo%20para%20el%20siglo%2021..pdf

[25] LONDON, Silvia and María Marta FORMICHELLA. Sen's concept of development and its link to education. Economy and Society [online]. 2006, XI(017), 17-32 [accessed: 11 November 2023]. ISSN 18070-414X. disponible en: https://ri.conicet.gov.ar/bitstream/handle/11336/131525/CONICET_Digital_Nro.e118e324-041c-482d-975d-512a59b6fd95_A.pdf?sequence=2&isAllowed=y

[26] HERNÁNDEZ GARZÓN, Yamile. The formation of informational competencies in university students. Case of the University of Bogotá Jorge Tadeo Lozano. [online]. Colombia, 2019 [accessed: 11 November 2023]. Master's thesis. Pontificia Universidad Javeriana. Available at: https://repository.javeriana.edu.co/bitstream/handle/10554/46136/Tesis_Maestría_en_Educación_Hernandez_Yamile.pdf?sequence=2&isAllowed=y

[27] MOIRA, Brent and Ruth STUBBINGS. The SCONUL Seven Pillars of Information Literacy. Core Model For Higher Education [online]. 2011 [cited: 21 May 2023]. Aviable: https://www.sconul.ac.uk/sites/default/files/documents/coremodel.pdf

[28] HERNÁNDEZ SAMPIERI, Roberto, Carlos FERNÁNDEZ COLLADO and Pilar BAPTISTA LUCIO. Metodología de la Investigación [online]. 6th ed. Mexico City: McGraw Hill, 2014 [accessed: 21 May 2023]. ISBN 978-1-4562-2396-0. Available at: https://www.uca.ac.cr/wp-content/uploads/2017/10/Investigacion.pdf

[29] JIMÉNEZ PUERTO, Carlos Lázaro and María de las Mercedes CALDERÓN MORA. Informational competence as a requirement for academic training in the 21st century. Gaceta Médica Espirituana [online]. 2020, 22(3), 147-159 [accessed: 21 May 2023]. ISSN 1608-8921. Available at: http://scielo.sld.cu/scielo.php?script=sci_arttext&pid=S1608-89212020000300147&nrm=iso

[30] ZAPE GRANDA, Sindy Dayana. Information literacy, reading and writing program for Higher Education Institutions [online]. Colombia, 2020 [accessed on October 10, 2023]. Undergraduate Thesis. Universidad Nacional Abierta y a Distancia UNAD. Available at: https://repository.unad.edu.co/handle/10596/38538

[31] HERNÁNDEZ CAMPILLO, Thais Raquel, Bárbara María CARVAJAL HERNÁNDEZ and María de los Ángeles LEGAÑOA FERRÁ. Analysis of informational competencies in the continuing education of university teachers. Libraries. Anales de Investigación [online]. 2020, 16(1), 61-69 [accessed. 07 October 2023]. ISSN 0006-176X. Available at: http://revistas.bnjm.sld.cu/index.php/BAI/article/view/47

[32] JIMÉNEZ PUERTO, Carlos Lázaro, María de las Mercedes CALDERÓN MORA yYaleidys CORRALES VALDIVIA. El proceso de formación, una mirada hacia las competencias informacionales. Pedagogy and Society [online]. 2020, 23(28), 51-75 [accessed: 07 October 2023]. Available at: http://revistas.uniss.edu.cu/index.php/pedagogia-y-sociedad/article/view/1075

[33] RAMÍREZ GRANELA, R and MM FERNÁNDEZ VALDÉS. Diagnosis of information literacy skills of the professionals of the National Library of Cuba. Bib.An.Inves [online]. 2019, 15(1), 68-82 [accessed: 02 September 2022]. Available at: http://revistas.bnjm.cu/index.php/BAI/article/view/114

[34] URIBE TIRADO, Álvaro and María PINTO MOLINA. The incorporation of information literacy in Iberoamerican university libraries. Comparative analysis based on information from their websites. An. Documentation [online]. 2013, 16(2) [accessed: 03 September 2022]. Available at: https://revistas.um.es/analesdoc/article/view/analesdoc.16.2.175541

[35] BARCELÓHIDALGO, MayreyDamilsy GÓMEZ PAZ. Information skills training based on designthinking: work experience at the University of Cienfuegos, Cuba. Palabra Clave (La Plata) [online]. 2022, 12(1), e167 [accessed: 07 October 2023]. Available at: doi:10.24215/1853991212e167.

[36] ANCHONDOGRANADOS, Rocío, Javier TARANGO ORTIZ, Jesús CORTÉS VERA and Juan Daniel MACHIN MASTROMATTEO. Definition of standards in informational competencies in scientific communication and their application in Mexican university teachers. Anales de Documentación [online]. 2020, 23(2) [accessed: 21 May 2023]. ISSN 1697-7904. Available at: doi:10.6018/analesdoc.379381.

[37] TISCAREÑO, Ma. Lourdes, Javier TARANGO and Jesús CORTÉSVERA. Development of informational competencies in Hispanic American universities: theoretical foundations for a comprehensive assessment model. e-Information Science [online]. 2015, 6(1), 1-33 [accessed: 21 May 2023]. Available at: doi:10.15517/eci.v6i1.21826.

[38] QUINDEMIL TORRIJO, Eneida María. From competencies to informational competencies. Reflexiones sobre la formación por competencias en el ámbito académico. Contributions to the Social Sciences [online]. 2011, 13 [accessed: 21 May 2023]. Available at: https://www.eumed.net/rev/cccss/13/emqt.html

[39] GONZÁLEZ GARCÍA, Tania Rosa. Model for the development of research competencies with interdisciplinary approach in Health Technology [online]. Havana, 2017 [accessed: 27 July 2023]. Doctoral Thesis. University of Medical Sciences of Havana. Available at: https://tesis.sld.cu/index.php?P=DownloadFile&Id=449

[40] Bulletin of the Spanish Federation of Associations of Archivists, Librarians, Archaeologists, Museologists and Documentalists. 2008, LVIII(3). ISSN 02104164.

[41] MERSTENS, L. Management by labor competence in business and vocational training. 1998.

[42] AUSTRALIAN AND NEW ZEALAND INSTITUTE FOR INFORMATION LITERACY ELEARNING. Information Literacy Standards. [online]. B.m.: Australian and New Zealand Institute for Information Literacy elearning. 2004 [accessed: 27 July 2023]. Available at: http://www.aab.es/pdfs/gtbunormas08.pdf

[43] JIMÉNEZROJO, Ángel. Informational competence and critical thinking in non-university education: a systematic review. RiiTE Revista Interuniversitaria de Investigación en Tecnología Educativa [online]. 2020, (9) [accessed: 27 March 2023]. Available at: doi:10.6018/riite.431381.

[44] EISENBERG, Michael B, Janet MURRAY and Colet BARTOW. BIG6 by the month: a common sense approach to effective use of common standards for information literacy learning. Library Media Connection [online]. 2014, 32(6) [cited: 21 May 2023]. Aviable: https://www.proquest.com/docview/1550993651

[45] The 8Ws of Lamb OSLA [online]. 2019 [accessed: 21 May 2023]. Available from: http://www.bmns.sld.cu/declaraciones-modelos-y-normas

[46] SMALL, MC, ME PÉREZ and R ALVARADO. Models for the organization of the information search process (Alfin). Original Pedagogical Studies. 2017, Pedagogy Special.

[47] FERNÁNDEZ VALDÉS, María de las Mercedes and Roberto ZAYAS MUJICA. Informational competencies as a determinant for the equitable use of scientific information and technology in health. Bibliotecas. Research Annals [online]. 2016, 12(1) [accessed: 21 May 2023]. ISSN 0006-176X. Available at: http://revistas.bnjm.cu/index.php/BAI/article/view/162

[48] CUEVAS, A. Reading, information literacy and school library. Spain: Ediciones Trea, 2007.

[49] ANGULO MARCIAL, Noel. Normas de competencias en información. BiD: Textos unirsitaris de biblioteconomia i documentació [online]. 2003, 11(10) [accessed: 21 May 2023]. Available at: https://bid.ub.edu/11angul2.htm

[50] OLAZABAL GUERRA, Daniel José. Information Literacy. In: Competencias Informacionales y Entornos Colaborativos en Red. 2022.

[51] ZELADA PÉREZ, Malena. Information Literacy. In: Competencias Informacionales y Entornos Colaborativos en Red. 2020.

[52] CONGRESS OF COLOMBIA. Law 1341 [online]. July 30, 2009 [accessed: 02 August 2023]. Available at: https://mintic.gov.co/portal/inicio/Normatividad/Leyes/

[53] NATIONAL MEDICAL LIBRARY OF CUBA. What are ICT? National Medical Library [online]. 2023 [accessed: 02 August 2023]. Available at: http://www.bmns.sld.cu/que-son-las-tic

[54] BELLOCH ORTÍ, Consuelo. Las Tecnologías de la Información y Comunicación (T.I.C.) [online]. B.m.: Educational Technology Unit. Universidad

de Valencia. 2023 [accessed: 02 August 2023]. Available at: https://www.uv.es/~bellochc/pdf/pwtic1.pdf

[55] DOCUSIGN COLLABORATOR. What are ICTs, their advantages and examples to incorporate in your business. DocuSign [online]. 10 October 2022. [accessed: 02 August 2023]. Available at: https://www.docusign.mx/blog/TICs

[56] UNIVERSIDAD LATINA DE COSTA RICA. What are ICTs and what are they for? Universidad Latina de Costa Rica [online]. July 9, 2020 [accessed: August 02, 2023]. Available at: https://www.ulatina.ac.cr/articulos/que-son-las-tic-y-para-que-sirven

[57] COBO ROMANÍ, Juan Cristóbal. The concept of information technologies. Benchmarking on the definitions of ICT in the knowledge society. zer [online]. 2009, 14(27), 295-318 [accessed: 02 August 2023]. ISSN 1137-1102. Available at: https://addi.ehu.es/bitstream/handle/10810/40999/2636-8482-1-PB.pdf?sequence=1&isAllowed=y

[58] FERNÁNDEZ MUÑOZ, Ricardo. Conceptual framework of new technologies applied to education. [online]. 2015 [accessed: 02 August 2023]. Available is: http://www.uclm.es/profesorado/ricardo/DefinicionesNNTT. html.

[59] PIMENTEL, Ramón. Las Tics, its origin-evolution and contributions to education. Sutori [online]. 2023 [accessed: 12 August 2023]. Available at: https://www.sutori.com/es/historia/las-tics-su-origen-evolucion-y-aportes-a-la-educacion--gpWHGu1ahY1FSw9PVu416db7

[60] MANSO PEREA, César, Aurora CUEVAS CERVERÓ and Sergio GONZÁLEZ-CERVANTES. Informational competencies in undergraduate nursing studies: the Spanish case. Spanish Journal of Scientific Documentation [online]. 2019, 42(1), e229 [accessed: 26 March 2023]. Available at: doi:10.3989/redc.2019.1.1578.

[61] ÁLVAREZ CADAVID, Gloria María and César Augusto GONZÁLEZ MANOSALVA. Apropiación de TIC en docentes de la educación superior: una mirada desde los contenidos digitales. Praxis Educativa [online]. 2022, 26(1), 1-25 [accessed on March 26, 2023]. ISSN 2313-934X. Available at: doi:https://doi.org/10.19137/praxiseducativa-2022-260104

[62] CALLÍS FERNÁNDEZ, Sureima, Omara Margarita GUARTON ORTIZ, Virgen CRUZ SÁNCHEZ, Ada María DE ARMAS FERRERA, Ibis RUIZ GUERRERO and Gilberto QUEVEDO FREITES. Informational competences in teachers of the Josué País García Polyclinic. In: EDUMED Holguín 2019: VIII Jornada Científica de la SOCECS [online]. 2019, [accessed: 26 March 2023]. Available at: http://edumedholguin2019.sld.cu/index.php/2019/2019/paper/view/233/154

[63] ALONSO VAZQUEZ, Ariadna Victoria, Daylin Elizabeth GONZÁLEZ GARCÍA, Ismael DESPAIGNE DESPAIGNE, Alexander RODRÍGUEZ PORTALES, Leonor MÉNDEZ LEYVA yIday MATEO GONZÁLEZ. Informational competencies in the professionals of the Gynecobstetric Teaching

Hospital in Palma Soriano, Cuba. EDUMECENTRO [online]. 2021, 13, 147-161 [accessed on March 26, 2023]. ISSN 2077-2874. Available at: http://scielo.sld.cu/scielo.php?script=sci_arttext&pid=S2077-28742021000300147&nrm=iso

[64] CHAVEZ VILLADEAMIGO, Liliana and Liana GONZÁLEZ LIESEGANG. Informe del estado del arte de la implementación de Formación en Competencias Informacionales en la currícula de grado y/o en la educación permanente para Facultad de Derecho - Udelar [online]. Working Paper No. 3. Montevideo: Udelar. 2019 [accessed: 10 October 2023]. Available at: http://eprints.rclis.org/38950/

[65] MACHADO RAMÍREZ, Evelio Felipe and Nancy MONTES DE OCA RECIO. La formación por competencias y los vacíos del diseño curricular. Transformación [online]. 2021, 17, 459-478 [accessed: 10 October 2023]. ISSN 2077-2955. Available at: http://scielo.sld.cu/scielo.php?script=sci_arttext&pid=S2077-29552021000200459&nrm=iso

[66] VALVERDE GRANDAL, Orietta and Sol Angel ROSALES REYES. Proposal of a program for the formation of informational competences in undergraduate students of Stomatology. Cuban Journal of Stomatology [online]. 2017, 54(1) [accessed 10 October 2023]. ISSN ISSN 0034-7507. Available at: http://scielo.sld.cu/scielo.php?script=sci_arttext&pid=S0034-75072017000100001

[67] SUÁREZ JORGE, Alinoet. Theoretical-methodological conception for information literacy in preparation for employment in the career of Computer Science at the UCI. Havana, 2023. Doctoral Thesis. Technological University of Havana "José Antonio Echeverría", CUJAE.

[68] ESTRADA MOLINA, Odiel, Dieter Reynaldo FUENTES CANCELL and Willian SIMÓN GRASS. Formation of informational competencies in Bioinformatics from undergraduate studies at the University of Informatics Sciences. Cuban Journal of Health Sciences Information [online]. 2021, 32[accessed 10 October 2023]. ISSN 2307-2113. Available at: http://scielo.sld.cu/scielo.php?script=sci_arttext&pid=S2307-21132021000200010&nrm=iso

[69] AÑORGA MORALES, Julia, Dora L. ROBAU, G. MAGAZ and E. CABALLERO. CABALLERO. Glossary of Advanced Education Terms. Havana: ISPEJV. 2010, 48.

[70] VIRTUAL HEALTH CLASSROOM. Parameterization. Assisted Tutorial Doctorate in Medical Education Sciences [online]. [accessed. 12 September 2023]. Available at: https://aulavirtual.sld.cu/mod/glossary/showentry.php?eid=553

[71] LAZO, M. Interventive improvement strategy with an interdisciplinary approach for the improvement of the professional pedagogical performance of general comprehensive teachers. Havana, 2007. Doctoral Thesis. Enrique José Varona Higher Pedagogical Institute.

[72] ARTILES VISBAL, Leticia, Jacinta OTERO IGLESIAS and Irene BARRIOS OSUNA. Research Methodology for Health Sciences. Havana: Editorial Ciencias Médicas. 2009, 65-78.

[73] CAMPISTROUS, Luis and Celia RIZO. Indicadores e investigación educativa. Havana: Instituto Central de Ciencias Pedagógicas de Cuba. 1998.

[74] LORENZO PÉREZ, Milene Beatriz. Methodological Strategy for the Management of Statistical Information in the Implementation of the Mother and Child Program in Camagüey. Camagüey, 2019. Master's Thesis. University of Medical Sciences of Camagüey.

[75] BORGES OQUENDO, Lourdes de la Caridad. Model of Impact Evaluation of the academic postgraduate in teachers of the Faculty of Medical Sciences "General Calixto García" [online]. Havana, 2014 [accessed: 17 September 2023]. Doctoral dissertation. Enrique José Varona University of Pedagogical Sciences. Available at:
https://docs.bvsalud.org/biblioref/2018/06/884915/2014_borges_modelo_impacto_posgrado.pdf

[76] GONZÁLEZ GONZÁLEZ, Daniel and Norberto VALCÁRCEL IZQUIERDO. Evaluación y Acreditación Institucional. B.m.: Universidad Mayor, Real y Pontificia de San Francisco Xavier de Chuquisaca. Sucre, Bolivia: Centro de Estudios de Postgrado e Investigación. 2001

[77] SUÁREZ, Jennyffer, Denesy PALACIOS and Joffre VERA. Model of Methodological Strategies for the optimization of pedagogical processes. Encuentros [online]. 2023, (17), 77-90 [accessed: 17 September 2023]. ISSN 2343-6131.   Available   at:
http://encuentros.unermb.web.ve/index.php/encuentros/article/view/379/335

[78] ORTIZ QUIZHPI, EM. Implementation of methodological strategies based on cooperative work to enhance attention to the diversity of learning styles. Illari [online]. 2019, 1(7), 38-44 [accessed: 02 October 2023]. ISSN 1390-4485. Available at: https://revistas.unae.edu.ec/index.php/illari/article/view/305/257

[79] MAGALLÁN JIMÉNEZ, F, A FRANCO CASTRO and M TOBAR BOHÓRQUEZ. Methodological and innovative strategies in strengthening the geopolitics of Ecuador in university students. Reciamuc [online]. 2019, 2(1), 342-374 [accessed: 29 September 2023]. ISSN 2588-0748. Disponible en: https://doi.org/10.26820/reciamuc/2.1.2018.342-374

[80] AGUILAR-GORDÓN, F. The methodological proposal as an alternative for the integration of knowledge. Revista Cátedra [online]. 2019, 2(2), 94-110 [accessed: 01 October 2023]. ISSN 2631-2875. Available at: https:// doi.org/10.29166/catedra.v2i2.1708.

[81] MERO LINO, Edwin Antonio, María Mercedes ORTIZ HERNÁNDEZ a KleberGerminiano MARCILLO PARRALES. Methodological strategy for the development of digital competencies of university teachers in Ecuador. Serie Científica Universidad de las Ciencias Informáticas [online]. 2023, 16(9), 177-184

[accessed: 22 September 2023]. ISSN 2306-2495. Available at: https://publicaciones.uci.cu/index.php/serie/article/view/1438

[82] SUAREZ JORGE, Alinoet. Theoretical-methodological conception for information literacy in preparation for employment in Computer Science. In: V International Scientific Convention UCIENCIA 2023. Electronic presentation. Varadero, Matanzas, Cuba. September 28, 2023.

[83] VALLE LIMA, Alberto D. Pedagogical research. Otra mirada. Havana: Pueblo y Educación, 2012. ISBN 978-959-13-2263-0.

[84] VIGOSTKI, L. S. Thought and language. Revolutionary Edition. B.m.: Pueblo y Educación, 1968.

[85] CHÁVEZ, J and OTHERS. Necessary approach to General Pedagogy. 2005.

[86] PROFUTURO. ICT competencies for teachers according to UNESCO. ProFuturo [online]. 3 August 2022. [accessed: 22 September 2023]. Available at: https://profuturo.education/observatorio/competencias-xxi/competencias-tic-para-docentes-segun-unesco/

[87] MUJICA-SEQUERA, Ruth M. Technological Trends 2022. Docentes 2.0 [online]. 21 December 2021 [accessed: 11 November 2023]. Available at: https://blog.docentes20.com/2021/12/%E2%9C%8Dtendencias-tecnologicas-2022-docentes-2-0/

[88] MUJICA-SEQUERA, Ruth M. Technological Trends in Education 2023. Docentes 2.0 [online]. 21 June 2023 [accessed: 11 November 2023]. Available at: https://blog.docentes20.com/2023/06/%e2%9c%8dinfografia-tendencias-tecnologicas-en-la-educacion-2023-docentes-2-0/

[89] ESCOBAR PÉREZ, Jazmine a CUERVO MARTÍNEZ. Content validation and expert judgment: an approach to their use. Advances in Measurement [online]. 2008, 6, 27-36 [accessed: 10 October 2023]. Available at: https://www.humanas.unal.edu.co/lab_psicometria/application/files/9416/0463/3548/Vol_6._Articulo3_Juicio_de_expertos_27-36.pdf

[90] TRAN, Astrid. 40 best Likert scale examples | Updated 2023. AhaSlides [online]. 10 November 2023 [accessed: 11 November 2023]. Available at: https://ahaslides.com/es/blog/likert-scale-examples/

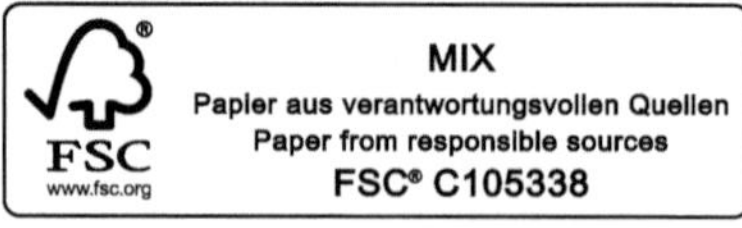

Printed by Books on Demand GmbH, Norderstedt / Germany